LUNCH BUDDIES

Buddy Up for a Better Diet

Lynette Fleming
Susan Dudra

Copyright © 2008 by Lynette Fleming

All rights reserved. Printed in the United States of America. No part of this publication may be reproduced, stored in a retrieval system, or transmitted in any form or by any means, electronic, mechanical, photocopying, recording, or otherwise, without the written permission of the authors.

ISBN 978-0-578-00136-4

Our deepest gratitude to:

My sister, Cindy Tieken, for creating the illustration on our book cover, and for allowing us to talk about her medical condition.

Nancy Moffett, retired Assistant Metro Editor of the Chicago Sun Times, for her encouragement and editing assistance.

Mickey Gaines, owner of Broadway Bazaar Costumes in Mt. Zion, Illinois, for her expert assistance in selecting the costumes used to depict the history of the foods highlighted in each chapter of this book.

Doug Miller, owner of Millers Studio of Photography in Mt. Zion, Illinois, who photographed most of the pictures contained within this book.

To our families who supported us, patiently listened to us, watched us cooking, tried our recipes, and gave us suggestions as we researched and wrote this book.

This book can be purchased at the websites of Lulu, Barnes & Noble, Amazon, and Books a Million. Web: *www.lunchbuddiesdiet.com*

Table of Contents

Table of Contents _____ *i*

Culinary Time Travel _____ *1*

Raw Foods Fit for Royalty _____ *19*

    Facts and Folklore _____ 29

    Balsamic Strawberry Salad _____ 66

    Black Bean and Wild Rice Salad _____ 68

    Black Bean Salsa Salad _____ 69

    Citrus/Mango Salad with Toasted Walnuts _____ 70

    Cucumber and Carrot Salad _____ 71

    Dr. Weil's Citrus Dressing _____ 72

    Gil's Salad _____ 73

    Grapefruit and Avocado Salad _____ 74

    Lentil & Garbanzo Bean Salad _____ 75

    Lunch Buddy Salad _____ 76

    Lunch Buddy Fruit Salad _____ 77

    Lunch Buddy Pasta Salad _____ 78

    Melon Salad with Mint and Honey _____ 80

    O Baby! Greens _____ 81

    Vinaigrettes _____ 81

    Pepper Salad _____ 82

    Red and Green Salad _____ 83

    Red Wine Vinaigrette _____ 83

    Romaine and Pear Salad with Walnuts and Chive Flowers _84

Table of Contents

- Spinach Fennel Salad with Oranges — 85
- Sweet as Dessert Salad — 86
- Strawberry Spinach Salad — 88
- Tomato Cucumber Salad — 89
- Triple Berry Salad — 90
- Nuts — 91

Heavenly Herbs and Spices — *93*

The Magic Mushroom — *113*

- Cream of Mushroom Soup with Quinoa — 117
- Fettucine with Shiitake Mushrooms — 118
- Hot and Sour Soup — 120
- Mushroom Barley Soup — 121
- Mushrooms with Garlic — 123
- Mushroom and Spinach Frittata — 124
- Mushroom and Vegetable Soup — 125
- Pasta with Cremini — 126
- Porcini Risotto — 129
- Wild Rice and Mushroom Soup — 131

Go Go Grains — *133*

- Barley and Lentil Stew with Mushrooms — 146
- Barley Stuffed Bell Peppers — 147
- Confetti Rice — 148
- Hearty Barley Soup — 149
- Mushroom Barley Bake — 150
- Mushroom Rice Bake — 151

Table of Contents

- Quinoa Pilaf _____ 152
- Roasty Toasty Barley Stew _____ 153
- Summer Garden Quinoa _____ 155
- Tomato Oatmeal Soup _____ 156
- Vegetarian Chili with Brown Rice _____ 157
- Wild Rice and Mushrooms _____ 159
- Wild Rice, Pine Nuts and Cranberries _____ 160

The Beneficent Bean... _____ *163*

- Black Bean and Corn Casserole _____ 169
- Black Bean Vegetable Soup _____ 171
- Creole Beans and Brown Rice _____ 172
- Crockpot Bean Soup _____ 174
- Italian Bean Soup _____ 175
- Lentil, Barley and Bacon Soup _____ 176
- Lunch Buddy Freezer Wraps _____ 177
- Penne with a Punch _____ 179
- Provencal Bean Soup _____ 180
- Red Lentil Soup _____ 181
- South of the Border Garlic Vegetable Soup _____ 182
- Tomato, White Bean, and Yellow Squash Stew _____ 183
- Two Bean and Rice Bake _____ 185
- Vegetarian Chili _____ 186
- White Bean Fennel Soup _____ 188

Pasta Promotion _____ *191*

- Angel Hair with Fresh Herbs and Roma Tomatoes _____ 196

Table of Contents

Couscous with Cabbage and Mushrooms ___ 197
Marinara Sauce ___ 198
Orange Sesame Couscous ___ 199
Orzo and Mushrooms with Edamame ___ 200
Penne with Roasted Chickpeas, Peppers and Spinach ___ 201
Roasted Roma Penne Pasta ___ 202
Spaghetti with Sun-dried Tomatoes and Peas ___ 204
Tomatoes Stuffed with Vegetable Couscous ___ 205
Walnut Pasta Toss ___ 206
Whole Wheat Pasta with Asparagus and Mushrooms ___ 207
Whole Wheat Pasta with Fresh Herbs ___ 209

Versatile Vegetable Hot Recipes ___ *211*

Baked Sweet Potato Slices with Herbs ___ 212
Broccoli with Lemon and Dill ___ 213
Fabulous Four-Veggie Roast ___ 214
Healing Cabbage Soup ___ 215
Herbed Asparagus with Parmesan Cheese ___ 216
Moroccan Vegetable Ragout ___ 217
Oven Roasted Autumn Vegetables ___ 219
Raw Roast ___ 220
Red Cabbage with Apple ___ 221
Roasted Asparagus with Gruyere ___ 222
Roasted Beets ___ 223
Roasted Ratatouille ___ 224
Stuffed Sweet Peppers ___ 225
Tomato Cabbage Soup with Barley ___ 226

Ultimate Vegetable Soup ___227
Zucchini and Tomato Casserole ___229

Quick and Easy Recipes ___ *231*

Lunch Buddy Sandwich Wraps ___232
Quick and Easy Garlic Bread ___233
Roasted Red Pepper Hummus ___234
Steve's Mango Salsa ___235
Steve's Salsa ___235

Tips and Tools ___ *237*

Lunch Buddy Rules ___242
Necessary Kitchen Gadgets ___249
Sample Menu ___253
Lunch Buddy Shopping List ___254
Foods High in Total Antioxidant Capacity (TAC) ___256

References and Recommended Resources ___ *258*

Index ___ *263*

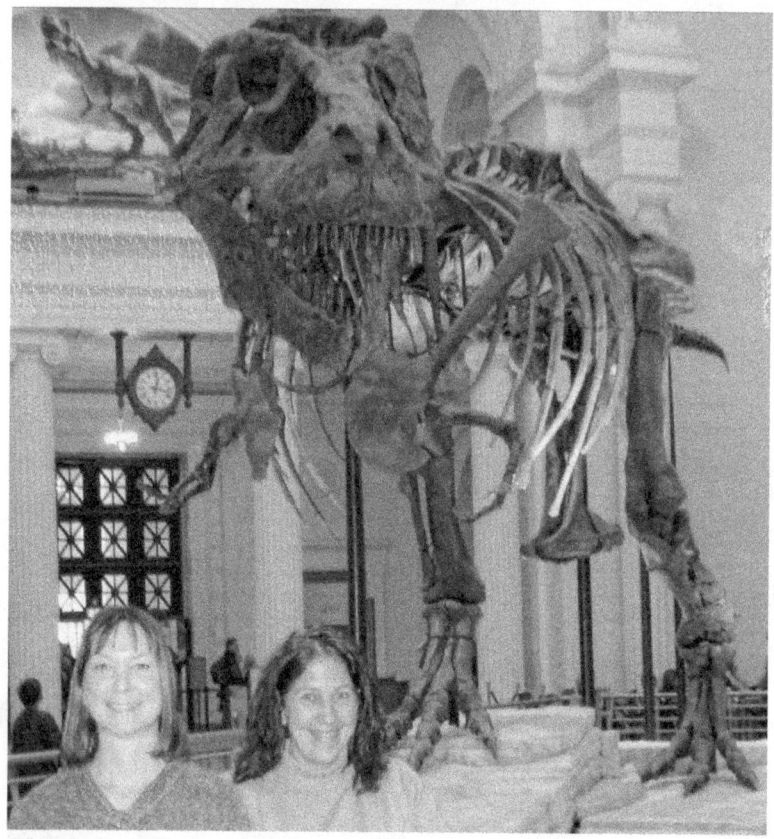

Photo 1 – We are going to take you on a trip to learn about the world's healthiest foods, many of which have been around for thousands and thousands of years. Some date back to the very first civilization, and some may even have been gobbled up by Sue's cousins, the Herbivores. We asked, but she's not talking.

Photo taken at the Field Museum of Natural History in Chicago, Illinois.

Culinary Time Travel

Whether you go to the bookstore, the grocery store, search online, or even check out your own cookbook collection, you will find numerous "healthy" cookbooks. You'll find cookbooks by associations, such as the American Diabetes Association, Weight Watchers, and the American Heart Association. You'll find books by movie stars, their trainers, physicians, dietitians, and a multitude of other famous people.

So you might ask yourself, "Why do I need this book?" The answer is simple. Because the authors are **not** actresses, models, dietitians, or physicians ... we are two ordinary middle-age women who (like many of you), are married to ordinary overweight, meat-loving men, with families who don't care for whole wheat anything. We go to work every day in a department which celebrates birthdays and holidays with a food day and a boss who keeps candy bars in a little bowl on his desk.

Our food days are to die for, with the cooks proudly marching in with their favorite fattening dishes and the non-cooks offering up bags of chips and dip, salsa, or donuts. The bakers tote in their favorite cakes, cookies, or brownies, and we eat all day from 8:00 am to 5:00 pm. We go home to our hungry families so full we can barely look at the food we have to cook. Sound familiar?

Susan and I have worked for our local hospital a combined total of 65 years. Susan worked in several departments before transferring to Human Resources, where I have worked as a recruiter since graduating from the School of Business at the University of Illinois in 1979. Although we didn't really know each other before her transfer, we have a lot in common. In addition to husbands who make it difficult to eat right at home, we each had quite a few grand years of eating whatever we wanted without paying for it later. Then came the middle age metabolism slow-down.

For several years, we coped in different ways. Susan called a small yogurt at her desk lunch, while I went to the cafeteria or coffee shop with my former "lunch buddies," who have since retired or found other jobs. I carefully selected a protein, a carbohydrate, and a vegetable. Then I walked past the desserts, and usually one would catch my eye. My favorite, strawberry shortcake ... "I'm eating right ... it won't hurt to add this small dessert," I'd say to myself. And then one day while shopping for clothes, I realized the ugly truth. Looking in the two-way mirror I murmured under my breath, "How did my rear get so big?" In addition to the problem with what used to be my cute little butt, I also had a digestive disorder, which I self-diagnosed as irritable bowel syndrome. On top of the digestive disorder, I now believe I was experiencing episodes with my gall bladder whenever I ate fatty foods or too much food, based on the fact that my mom, aunt, and sister have all had gall bladder surgery.

So the very next day on my way home from work, I stopped by the book store and bought the <u>Better Homes and Gardens New Dieter's Cookbook</u>. I planned a new meal every day for a week. My son helped with some of the preparation and was a pretty good sport about trying these new recipes. However, at the end of the week my husband handed me **his** list of favorite foods. He thought that I had forgotten his favorites (early Alzheimer's maybe?) ... pork chops, steak, spaghetti, fried chicken, tacos, etc. Goodbye diet.

4   Culinary Time Travel

How could I eat right with a husband unwilling to give up his favorite fattening foods? I tried making different meals for each of us. It's a great concept, but not very practical for a working mother. How could I possibly find the time to prepare an extra meal when I needed to help a son with his homework, pay the bills, do the laundry, clean the floors, go to work, and exercise regularly? Susan faced nearly the same hurdles at home, minus the son still at home. Like me, she also had some digestive problems, and was taking fiber pills for regularity.

I decided to focus on a healthy lunch since dinner wasn't going so well. I didn't want to eat lunch out of a cardboard box by myself. So one day I brought in two "Make Ahead Lunch Wraps," a recipe I found on *www.allrecipes.com*, and I asked Susan to join me for lunch. To my surprise, she said, "Sure." The next day we had lunch wraps again, and Susan brought a salad. The rest is history. We decided to become "lunch buddies" every day, each bringing a healthy dish (or dishes) to share.

After finishing our lunch, we would plan our meal for the next day. Make a spinach salad with fresh oranges, and then toss in a few walnuts. Make Andrew Weil's citrus

Culinary Time Travel

salad dressing. Nibble on blueberries for dessert ... or blackberries, raspberries, or apples. Make a recipe with barley, lentils, brown rice, or couscous. Make a split pea soup or vegetable soup from scratch using our favorite vegetables.

Within a few months our stomach and intestinal problems were gone, and we felt better than ever before. One night, before I fell asleep, it came to me. We should write a book, which would help thousands of other people just like us. The next day I asked Susan what she thought. She agreed it was a great idea!

To test the publishing waters, we wrote to Arlene Mannlein, a writer for the Life section of our local newspaper, and invited her to join us for a "lunch buddy" lunch. To our delight (and hers), she accepted. She loved the dishes we prepared, and our story appeared on the front page of the Life section. Everywhere we went, people began to ask when our book would be available.

That's our story ... now let's talk about you. Why should you recruit a lunch buddy? Have you ever read that it is best to exercise with a friend? Why not apply that principle to lunch? Find a lunch buddy or form your own

Culinary Time Travel

lunch club and you will inspire, motivate, and encourage each other. You each prepare a dish to share, saving calories, money, and time.

Let's talk about saving calories first. Here's a quote we found on *www.webmd.com* in "Brown-Bag Lunches That Make the Grade" by Barbara Russi Sarnataro. "The more home-cooked meals you have, the better," says WebMD Weight Loss Clinic "Recipe Doctor" Elaine Magee, MPH, RD. "Studies have shown that when people eat meals away from home, they eat more food, more calories and more fat."

What about time? The time you spend driving to lunch, standing in line, or waiting to be served adds up. Think what you could do with that extra time ... reading, working out, walking, or surfing (the internet, of course).

Now, money. Bill Ward states in a September 22, 2008 newspaper article titled "Workers save by bringing bagged lunches," "Whether brown bagging or dining at the office café, employees are scaling back on lunch costs. And the savings can add up quickly." Investment and personal-finance firms such as Family Credit Management and Bankrate.com estimate that workers can save $70 per month based on 20 meals with an average cost of $3.00 for a

Culinary Time Travel

'brown-bag' vs. $6.50 for a purchased meal. By the time you add in a tip and the cost of gas, that $840.00 annual savings will turn into more than $1,000.00. And for those of you who live in the city, the cost of your meal is probably a whole lot more than $6.50. On one website we found pitching the brown bag lunch, the author claims she is saving $3,000.00 a year by preparing her own lunch.

Now here's a bonus you may not have thought of. Anybody ever reach into the produce compartment of your refrigerator and grab a slimy surprise? If just one of you buys the green onions, chances are they'll be used before they turn into slime. By planning your lunches and sharing with your buddy, you'll be able to use your produce while it's still fresh. Best of all, unlike the small, tasteless meals out of cardboard boxes, this food is delicious, filling, and is actually good for you.

We have created and enjoyed every recipe in this book, some of which are a more healthy variation of a recipe found in another book or on a website. We have made it easy for you to incorporate our recipes and others like them into your diet. You will begin your day on a healthy note, taking in a variety of vitamins, minerals, whole grains, and fiber before your afternoon break. You'll soon forget about the candy bars, chips, and pop.

Some of you may have read (or heard of) The Dorm Room Diet, written by Daphne Oz for the thousands of college students who find it difficult to eat right. Some may have read Skinny Bitch, written by Rory Freedman and Kim Barnouin, appealing especially to any woman belonging to Generation X or Generation Y. People who are serious about dieting have probably read The Sonoma Diet, by Dr. Connie Guttersen. Intelligent people who want to understand the science behind good nutrition have probably read every Dr. Andrew Weil book, including Eating Well for Optimum Health. We love all these books and recommend you read them, incorporating whatever ideas you can into your daily routine.

We were a little over halfway finished writing Lunch Buddies when my 15-year-old son, Michael, saw me reading Skinny Bitch. As a normal teenage boy, he wanted to know if the authors were cute. I handed him the book, he quickly flipped it over, and a long low whistle ensued. "Mom, I really think you and Susan could sell more books if you looked like them," he said, not intending to hurt my feelings. "Honey," I replied, "Susan and I can't turn back the clock, so do you think we'd sell more if we renamed our book <u>Skinny Old Bitches</u>?" He laughed so hard, he nearly choked on his cheeseburger.

The truth is we aren't skinny, although we have both lost some weight since beginning <u>Lunch Buddies</u> in 2005. I've lost twelve pounds, Susan's lost six, and best of all we are not packing on the pounds like many of our post-menopausal friends. We are both within our recommended weight range, and we are doing everything we can to stay there. It's really pretty simple to do, as you'll soon learn.

When you're young (under 40), the primary goal of eating right is to improve your appearance. When you're over 40, you read the obituaries ... and suddenly you notice people your age and younger are actually dying. If that doesn't scare you into eating right, nothing will. We can't control time, but we can control what we put in our mouths.

If you're overweight, as nearly two-thirds of American adults are, you may be heading toward a disaster with your heart, your knees, your hips, and your quality of life. Women over 30 gain an average of 10 pounds per decade. That means that if you're already 10 pounds overweight at age 30, by the time you reach your 50's you'll be 30 pounds overweight. Those extra 30 pounds are going to wreak havoc on your body. Combining age and extra weight is a recipe for disaster. If you're already overweight, change your eating habits now, before the disaster. If your weight is fine, change your eating habits to maintain your weight and your good health.

You may think there isn't time in your morning routine to prepare lunch. We have done it, and we'll show you how. It's easier than you think. Our recipes are simple and delicious. The goal isn't really to lose weight, but to become healthier. And when you do, your weight will drop like raindrops on your head during a thunderstorm. Ok, maybe not that fast ... let's say slow and steady like a turtle crossing the field to get to the pond.

You may be tempted to eat our recipes for dinner. Great idea! However, if you eat a donut for breakfast, a whopper and fries for lunch, and then eat a lunch buddy recipe for dinner, you definitely won't be losing any weight. If you guzzle soda and gobble sweets throughout the day, you're on the fast train to Obesityville, no matter what you eat for dinner. You need to eat right beginning with your first step out of bed.

All you have to do is check out your local supermarket, and you will find food that is organic, free of trans-fats, low in calories, sodium and fat, or enriched with a variety of vitamins and minerals. How do you know what to buy and what to eat?

We recommend you stay away from diets which eliminate a food group. The key to a healthy diet is eating lots of fresh fruits and vegetables, whole grains, beans, and legumes. Eliminate or cut back on your meat consumption. Don't eat processed foods. Don't drink soda or other sugary drinks, or diet drinks. Do drink lots of water and tea, especially green tea (but not the kind with all the sugar in it). If you don't like water, toss in a slice of lemon or lime.

If losing weight fast is your goal, raw fruits and vegetables should comprise 75% of your diet. I did this once when I wanted to reduce quickly before a Caribbean cruise. I lost a pound or two a week and dropped eighteen pounds in three months. It's really easy to do in the summer when a variety of fresh produce is available. We have some fabulous raw food recipes you won't be able to resist.

Culinary Time Travel

Most of the foods you will be incorporating into your diet have been around for thousands of years. It wasn't until the late 1930's that processed foods became a staple in the American diet. A man named Clarence Birdseye, after an expedition to Labrador, developed the first frozen foods based on what he observed in the Arctic. By 1925 he was selling frozen fish fillets through his new company, the General Seafoods Company, which later expanded to include meats, poultry, fruits, and vegetables. Kraft introduced its first stovetop macaroni and cheese dinners, which included cheese sauce packets in 1937, just prior to the time when people in the United States were searching for foods to help them compensate for dairy rations and difficulty purchasing meat.

Some of you baby boomers may have memories like mine. Mom went back to work when my baby brother started kindergarten, and I was in third grade. One summer, after we got every one of our babysitters fired, Mom decided I was old enough to be the babysitter. I made our lunches out of a box or a can ... Chef Boyardee spaghetti, Kraft macaroni and cheese, pizza out of a box, hot dogs. These were convenient and easy meals for a young, inexperienced cook.

My maternal grandma, Myrtle Focht, was born in 1893. When she was a young girl, she fell out of a horse-drawn carriage on her way to church and the carriage ran over her. The doctor told her parents she probably wouldn't live to be much past 20.

Grandma Focht lived long past 20 and as a homemaker kept no boxed items in her cupboards. Every summer I got to stay with her a week, and every morning she made me homemade cinnamon rolls (from scratch, girls, not the frozen kind). She never bought a loaf of bread or stick of margarine. I loved eating her "real" bread and butter. She and my grandpa had a huge garden, including red raspberry and black raspberry bushes. We'd go out and eat the berries right off the bush. At the end of my visit, when Mom came to pick me up (and she still reminds me of this today), I cried because I didn't want to go home. (Sorry, Mom.) Grandma was a great cook, and I loved eating everything she made.

Grandma Focht never learned to drive, and after Grandpa died, she walked everywhere she needed to go.

Culinary Time Travel

Every summer, even in her 90's, she flew (by herself) from Lima, Ohio to Myrtle Beach, South Carolina to visit Mom. In her later years, the airlines always offered to get her a wheelchair, and she would tell them in quite a firm tone to save it for someone who needed it. In spite of the homemade cinnamon rolls, real butter, cooking with lard, and the doctors' predictions of her short life span, Grandma lived to be 99 ½, and never had to live in a nursing home. Proud of you, Grandma! I really don't know whether her long healthy life was due to genetics, to the lack of processed foods in her diet, to walking everywhere instead of driving, or all these factors, but I do know it is possible to cook with whole foods like grandma even if you work and that if you do, you will be all the healthier for it.

In this book, you will journey back thousands of years to learn some fascinating facts about foods. You may be surprised to learn that some of these foods were actually grown by the very first civilization more than 10,000 years ago. Some will bring back memories, like mine of picking berries with my grandma and helping her gather the eggs in the chicken house. What you will find is that these foods

Culinary Time Travel

which have been around for thousands of years are the very foods you **must** include in your diet.

While it's fun to look back at the history of these healthy foods, it's imperative to look back at your own family history, and the diseases and conditions to which you may be genetically predisposed. Has anyone died as a result of diabetes, heart disease, asthma, pneumonia, or cancer? Anyone suffered from arthritis, osteoporosis, gall bladder disease, or hypoglycemia? What you learn will help you determine which foods to eat, and which ones to avoid.

Diabetes is a problem in my family. My paternal grandfather, my dad, his two brothers, and my sister all are (or in some cases were) diabetic. Grandpa Sprang died at only 55 of a heart attack, likely brought on by the ravages of diabetes and a smoking habit. I've heard he was a great guy with a wonderful sense of humor, but I never had a chance to know him. I do remember looking up at the casket and my dad lifting me up to kiss him goodbye. Today dad is 78, a heart attack survivor with declining eyesight, and my sister has diabetes-related stomach problems. I have seen what diabetes can do, and I know I have a 33% chance of getting the disease. Mom has had a stroke, and my mom, my aunt, and my sister have had gall bladder disease. To reduce my risk factors for all these conditions and diseases, I need to stay within my recommended weight range, eat lots of fruits, vegetables, and whole grains, eat less meat, stay away from sweets and simple carbohydrates, and exercise regularly.

How many times have you heard people say, "You gotta die of something … might as well eat what I want, I'm gonna die anyway." Yes, everyone is going to die of something sometime. But wouldn't you rather die at 85 than 55? A little prevention, including healthy eating, may go a long way toward maintaining your good health well into your 80's and beyond.

While other diet books appeal to college students, meat lovers, meat haters, zealous dieters, and movie stars, <u>Lunch Buddies</u> may appeal most to the common working woman. The idea could certainly be helpful for housewives, couples, or even teens and schoolchildren, but women who work generally already have a lunch buddy which makes it just a matter of switching their diet from unhealthy processed foods to healthy unprocessed foods.

Culinary Time Travel

If Daphne Oz thinks it's difficult to eat right as a college student, just wait until she gets a job. Right, ladies? The workplace is like a minefield, with vending machines full of candy bars, chips, and pop around every corner. Many companies view vending as a profit center, not deducting the increased health costs associated with an overweight and obese workforce. Even if you manage to avoid the vending machines, if you go out to lunch you're probably going to eat the wrong foods and too much of them. The best and safest way to make sure you eat a healthy lunch is to bring your own, or better yet bring a healthy dish to share with a friend.

<u>Lunch Buddies</u> is like no other book or cookbook you've ever read. It capitalizes on friendship to achieve good health, and weaves a little history with a thread of humor about the healthiest of foods, most of which have been around for thousands of years. (Even longer than we have.) So get ready to travel back to a time when there were no processed foods, experience a little history, and enlighten your mind, your diet, and your body.

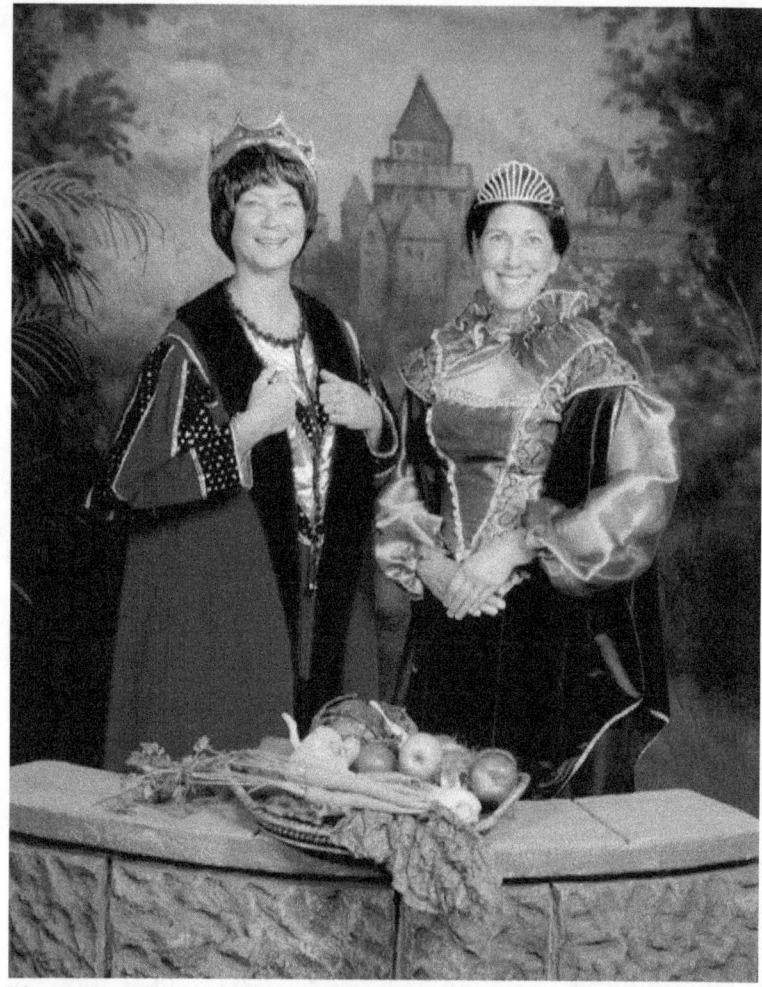

Photo 2 – Kings and Queens enjoyed a royal feast of the very best fruits and vegetables in the kingdom.

Raw Foods Fit for Royalty

Did your mother ever tell you to eat your vegetables? Of course she did because her mother said the same thing to her many, many years ago. Grandma knew the importance of fruits and vegetables, and grew most of her own produce in her own garden, tended to by grandpa and her nearly every day.

Whenever Susan eats beets, she fondly remembers the telltale tiny red juice lines around the corners of her grandma's mouth, proof that grandma enjoyed the beet juice as much as the beets themselves. My own grandma used every bit of her cabbage, and if I was lucky she'd share the cabbage heart with me. While our grandparents canned and froze their garden produce, our parents decided picking these items up at the supermarket was a lot more convenient. Most of the fruits and vegetables Susan and I grew up with were canned. Perhaps it was the same at your house.

Susan's family usually had a small garden so they could enjoy tomatoes and strawberries in the summertime. Other than that, most of the fresh foods she enjoyed were at grandma's house. Her grandma had apples and bananas on hand year-round and in the summer months she had squash, onions, peaches, blackberries, and beets (of course). "If Grandma were here today, I'd fix her my salad tossed with beet greens and watch her smile," Susan reminisced at lunch one day, "and maybe I'd be lucky enough to see the beet juice in the corners of her mouth." Susan's grandma may not have known the nutritional benefits of the foods she ate, but what she did know was very basic ... they tasted good!

While most people are aware that eating fruits, vegetables, nuts, and seeds is associated with a long, healthy life, they are not aware of the amazing nutritional value of each plant or seed. So let's talk a little bit about nutrition. Researchers tell us that plants are made up of more than 40,000 phytonutrients, the name given to the parts of plants that have health benefits. These phytonutrients are separated into groups, with each group having its own unique phytos and unique antioxidants.

Ever wonder why antioxidant levels aren't listed on food labels? Perhaps it's because researchers with the U.S. Department of Agriculture just recently were able to add the total amount of lipid-soluble and water-soluble antioxidant chemicals in foods to determine their Total Antioxidant Capacity (TAC). The chart on page 256 in the Tips and Tools chapter lists the best of the best, the foods we all should have on our team to defend us against the free radicals which cause some diseases, to prevent other diseases, and to delay the aging process. We found this chart in the fall 2008 issue of <u>Clean Eating</u> in a well-written and informative article, "Food TKO" by Matthew Kadey. Be sure to read it!

To make sure that you get the most nutritional value from your produce choices, you need to "eat the rainbow." The National Cancer Society, the American Cancer Society, and the Produce for Better Health Foundation all endorse a diet filled with colorful fruits and vegetables. That's because each color group has different phytonutrients and antioxidants, which benefit our health in different ways.

In general, the deeper the color of the fruit or vegetable, the greater is its nutritional value. For instance, spinach gives you eight times the vitamin C that iceberg lettuce offers. A ruby red grapefruit provides 25 times more vitamin A than a white grapefruit. However, each fruit and vegetable has a unique complement of vitamins, minerals, fiber, and phytonutrients ... so not only should we eat a variety of colors, we should also eat a variety within each color group.

Green fruits and vegetables contain potent phytochemicals, such as lutein and indoles, as well as other essential nutrients. This color group can help lower cancer risk, improve eye health, and keep bones and teeth strong. Fruits from this color group are: apples (green), avocados, grapes (green), honeydew, kiwifruit, limes, and pears (green). Vegetables include: artichokes, arugula, asparagus, beans (green), broccoli, broccoli rabe, Brussels sprouts, cabbage (Chinese), cabbage (green), celery, chayote squash, cucumbers, endive, greens (leafy), leeks, lettuce, okra, onions (green), peas (green or English, snow, sugar snap), peppers (green), spinach, watercress, and zucchini.

Red fruits and vegetables offer vitamin C, as well as lycopene, ellagic acid, and anthocyanins. Lycopene, a strong antioxidant, is found in tomatoes and other red fruits. Lycopene may help reduce the risk of heart disease and some forms of cancer. In addition, there is compelling evidence that lycopene can play a role in prostate cancer prevention. The color red helps to keep your blood pressure low, boost your heart health, improve memory function, promote urinary tract health, and protect you against some cancers. Fruits include: apples (red), cherries, cranberries, grapefruit (pink/red), grapes (red), oranges, pears (red), pomegranates, raspberries, strawberries, and watermelon. Vegetables include: beets, onions (red), peppers (red), potatoes (red), radicchio, radishes, rhubarb, and tomatoes.

Blue and purple fruits and vegetables contain varying amounts of health-promoting phytonutrients, such as polyphenols and anthocyanins. This color group packs a powerful antioxidant punch, offering extra protection against some types of cancer and urinary tract infections. Blue and purple produce may boost your brain health and vision. Fruits include: blackberries, blueberries, currants (black), elderberries, figs (purple), grapes (purple), plums, prunes, and raisins. Vegetables include: asparagus (purple), Belgian endive (purple), cabbage (purple), carrots (purple), eggplant, peppers (purple), and potatoes (purple-fleshed).

Orange and yellow fruits and vegetables offer antioxidants, vitamin C, and other phytonutrients, including carotenoids and bioflavonoids, which may help promote heart and vision health and a healthy immune system, as well as offering cancer prevention. Fruits include: apples (yellow), apricots, cantaloupe, cape gooseberries, figs (yellow), grapefruit, kiwifruit (golden), lemons, mangoes, nectarines, oranges, papaya, peaches, pears (yellow), persimmons, pineapple, tangerines, and watermelon (yellow). Vegetables include: beets (yellow), carrots, corn (sweet), peppers (yellow), potatoes (yellow), pumpkin, rutabagas, squash (butternut), squash (yellow summer), squash (yellow winter), sweet potatoes, and tomatoes (yellow).

White, tan, and brown fruits and vegetables contain phytonutrients, such as allicin, found in the onion family. They contribute to heart health by helping you maintain healthy cholesterol levels, and they may lower the risk of some types of cancer. Fruits include: bananas, dates, nectarines (white), peaches (white), and pears (brown). Vegetables include: cauliflower, corn (white), garlic, ginger, Jerusalem artichoke, jicama, kohlrabi, mushrooms, onions, parsnips, potatoes (white-fleshed), shallots, and turnips.

Many people understand that antioxidants are good for us, but don't fully understand why. To understand the value of antioxidants, you have to first understand oxidation. Oxidation is a natural part of how our living bodies work, but if the process gets out of hand it can put us at risk for many difficulties by damaging our cells. That's where antioxidants come into play. They apply the brakes to the oxidation process and help keep us healthier longer. By eating raw foods we can take advantage of the antioxidants and phytonutrients in them. Researchers have further found that these thousands of phytonutrients work for us better in combination than alone. That is, if we eat many of them together we get the greatest benefit.

Phytonutrients and antioxidants are just the beginning of the benefits you'll reap by adding raw foods to your daily diet. Living (raw) foods provide a maximum amount of energy for a minimal amount of effort. Studies have shown that raw foods have healing powers that can alleviate many illnesses and conditions, such as low energy, allergies, digestive disorders, weak immune system, high cholesterol, candida, obesity, and weight problems. Research has also shown that a person can prevent the body's healthy cells from turning into malignant cancerous cells by consuming mostly a raw food diet, including whole organic foods.

Many people believe they can eat whatever they want (in moderation), and get their vitamins and fiber in a pill, just as Susan did several years ago. As she approached 50, she noticed she was growing and not in a good way. Susan had been skinny all her life and didn't know how to lose weight. She read that fiber would fill you up and help with weight loss, so she bought some fiber pills.

What is fiber? Dietary fiber is the part of a plant which is indigestible, found only in plant foods, like fruits, vegetables, nuts, and grains. Soluble fiber helps lower cholesterol and blood sugar levels. Insoluble fiber has passive water-attracting properties which help increase bulk, soften stool, and shorten transit time through the intestinal tract. Fiber is helpful in the treatment and prevention of constipation, hemorrhoids, and diverticulitis. Diverticula are pouches of the intestinal wall that can become inflamed and painful. While in the past a low-fiber diet was prescribed for this condition, it is now known that a high-fiber diet gives better results once the inflammation has subsided.

The 2005 Dietary Guidelines for Americans recommends intake of 14 grams of fiber per 1,000 calories consumed. So, if you consume a 2500 calorie diet, you should eat approximately 35 grams of fiber per day. The typical American diet provides only 12 grams per day.

Getting back to those fiber pills, Susan now knows she added maybe two to four grams depending on how many she took each day. So if she consumed twelve grams of fiber per day through her basically unhealthy diet and topped it off with another two to four grams from her fiber pills, she still wasn't getting anywhere close to the fiber she needed. Many of you are probably doing the same thing. Turn that F in fiber into an A, and eat your fruits and vegetables. The best way to receive the maximum benefits from each type of fiber is to eat a variety of fiber-rich foods.

Susan saw someone on television recently who said, "We don't have to be fat, we just need to be educated." We would change that to "We don't have to be fat or unhealthy; we just need to be educated." We will show you how to enjoy the best foods nature has to offer, so you can begin achieving your best health now. If you don't remember anything else from this chapter, remember this. We feast with our senses first. Color is key.

Remember seeing your first rainbow? It seemed like a miracle. If you could only walk to the end, you may have thought (like I did) that you would surely find a treasure. The great news is that the treasure is right here under your nose in the rainbow of fruits and vegetables we can grow (or buy) and eat. Green, red, blue, purple, orange, yellow, white, tan, and brown fruits and vegetables offer a treasure of good nutrition in phytonutrients, antioxidants, and fiber. Eat the rainbow, and you will begin your journey to the miracle of good health and weight control.

Raw Foods Fit for Royalty

Facts and Folklore

You may recall reading that the Israelites complained bitterly about missing the garlic, onions, and leeks they'd left behind in Egypt. Luckily for us, BC travelers took the seeds of their beloved foods with them as they journeyed from place to place. Thanks to their efforts we have a wide variety of foods available to us today.

The evolution of farming has resulted in greater production, partly through the use of pesticides. According to the Environmental Working Group (EWG), a nonprofit environmental research organization based in Washington, DC, you can lower your pesticide exposure by almost 90 percent by avoiding conventional versions of the top 12 most contaminated fruits and vegetables.

The EWG "Dirty Dozen" list is in order of most-to-least contaminated. If you frequently eat one or more of these fruits or vegetables, try to buy these items organic whenever you can. Make a copy of the Lunch Buddy Shopping List on page 254 and take it with you to the grocery store to help you remember which fruits and vegetables to buy organic when possible.

While the best way to reap the health benefits of fruits and vegetables without exposing yourself to potentially harmful pesticides is to choose organic produce whenever possible, sometimes it isn't always possible or even necessary. Dr. Andrew Weil tells us that it's OK to buy non-organic varieties of some fruits and vegetables, which tend to contain the least amount of pesticides. These fruits and vegetables are also listed on the Lunch Buddy Shopping List. However, don't forget to remove dirt and bacteria by washing them thoroughly before eating or cooking.

It is best to wash vegetables and fruits just before you're ready to use them. Roll leafy greens in paper toweling and then store in a plastic bag in the crisper part of your refrigerator. Prolong their freshness by not sealing the bag.

Also, some of you may have read that fruit begins to lose nutrients once it is cut. While it's true some nutrients are lost, it isn't much. So you can make a big fruit salad to share with your lunch buddy and it will remain nutritious refrigerated for a few days.

Here's another tip, this one for helping fruit ripen. Dig out your big fruit bowl and put it in plain view, either on your table or on the counter. When you store fruits together they help each other ripen. We put pears in the bowl first, stems down, then our apples. By the time the apples are gone, the pears are ripe and juicy!

Apples

From the beginning, ancient man was enamored with fruit. No matter what his origin, stories about early man connect him to a garden of paradise filled with fruit trees. The stories center on the abundance of fruit, an irresistible temptation to eat it, and a terrible consequence once he has given in to the temptation. Remember the story of Adam and Eve? As it turns out they weren't the only ones tempted by fruit ... the Greek, Teutonic, and Celtic cultures had a similar story about fruit and early man.

The timeline of apples began around 8000 BC when nomadic hunters/gatherers invented agriculture. Desert apples spread from the forests of their origin in the Tien Shan mountains of eastern Kazakhstan throughout the civilized world as both trade and military expeditions began among these earliest civilizations. Excavations at Jericho in the Jordan Valley revealed remains of apples dated to 6500

BC. In the United States we're familiar with the stories of John Chapman, aka Johnny Appleseed.

Susan's ancestors, the Robinsons, settled in Decatur, Illinois, in the early 1830's. At that time you could buy a city lot for a hat. Imagine that! After purchasing some land, Amos Robinson "procured 100 apple trees and he and his boys set them out," according to a book in our local library, History of Macon County. In just a few short years, the trees were producing a big crop of apples. Amos loved his apple orchard so much that he was buried in the family burial plot in 1836 in the midst of the orchard he had set out a few years before.

I, too, have an apple story in my family history. When I was very young, my paternal grandparents had a large apple orchard behind their house. One beautiful autumn day, a sack of apples saved my dad's life. Dad had a nearly full large sack of apples slung over his shoulder, and was helping his folks by picking apples from the top of the apple trees. Sitting by my grandma, I cried out as I watched the ladder (and my dad) fall away from the tree. Fortunately he fell on the apples, which cushioned his fall and protected him from serious injury. After we realized he was not seriously injured, we teased him about trying to make applesauce the "easy" way.

Apples are hard workers for our bodies. The pectin they contain relieves constipation and helps get toxins out quickly, thus lowering cholesterol. Most of their fiber content is found in the peel, but a medium peeled apple will still give you around 2 1/2 grams or more. Because their fiber is both soluble and insoluble, they naturally reduce cholesterol. Apples are an excellent source of quercitin, a phytonutrient in the flavonoid family. Quercitin does its best work at getting rid of free radicals when it's boosted with vitamin C, which apples just happen to contain. At only 80 or so calories per apple they're a great portable snack. Pick your favorite from over 7,000 varieties!

Asparagus

Susan's daughter and son-in-law live on land that has been in his family for five generations. While her son-in-law, David, isn't sure exactly how long their asparagus patch has been growing, he remembers his parents going out to the farm each spring to cut the tender green shoots. Asparagus plants take a few years to grow spears, but after that they can produce for years. Originally from the

Mediterranean area, it's believed asparagus was eaten in ancient Egypt. Asparagus is very high in vitamin K, vitamin C, and folate. Folate is important for women of childbearing age because it protects against birth defects. Asparagus is a good source of dietary fiber and contains just 43 calories in one cup. Buy it fresh in the spring and try it in our Herbed Asparagus with Parmesan Cheese on page 216.

Avocado

Is it a fruit or is it a vegetable? It's a fruit that contains more protein than any other fruit. It's been called an alligator pear, so named because of its rough skin. Avocados help the body absorb carotenoids and lycopene, another reason to eat fruits and vegetables together. While one cup has 235 calories, its monosaturated fats help lower LDL, the bad cholesterol, and boost HDL, the good cholesterol. It's a good source of vitamins K, C, and B6, fiber, potassium, and folate. The avocado has its origins in Central and South America where it's been enjoyed since 8000 BC! Today Mexico is the top producer, and in the U.S. avocados are grown in California and Florida.

Because they turn bitter when cooked, they're best enjoyed raw but you can add them to already cooked dishes. You'll enjoy their velvety creaminess in our South of the Border Garlic Soup on page 182 and in our Grapefruit and Avocado Salad on page 74. Sprinkle with lemon juice to prevent the browning that occurs after cutting them.

Bananas

In 327 BC Alexander the Great and his army made note of bananas in the Philippines and India. They weren't introduced in the U.S. until later in the 19th century due to lack of transportation beyond coastal towns. After avocados, bananas are next in giving us high levels of potassium. If you take a diuretic for high blood pressure you lose potassium as you urinate. Eating bananas will help restore your potassium level, which is important for heart function. They also give you soluble fiber, manganese, vitamins C and B6, and calcium. Another great portable food, bananas deliver energy because of their fruit sugar content. Add them sparingly to salads and add them last because they can become soft and brown.

Beets

We especially like beets because you can eat the entire plant. The leafy greens on the top provide calcium, potassium, beta-carotene, and iron. Enjoy them in salads or steam with other greens. Grate some of the bulb into a salad and the beets will add such a wonderful sweetness you won't even need salad dressing. Make sure to add the grated beets right before serving or the whole salad will be red! Try our Roasted Beets on page 223 for a flavor surprise.

Prehistoric civilizations ate beet greens, but the ancient Romans were the first to eat the purple roots. During the Napoleon years beets were used for sugar. Beets, in fact, are higher in sugar than any other vegetable.

One cup of beets has only 74 calories but delivers folate, fiber, potassium, vitamin C, and manganese. Studies have found that beets can help protect our hearts and may help protect us from colon cancer. Speaking of the colon, don't be alarmed by the color you may see in your stool or urine after eating beets! It's just a harmless condition known as beeturia.

Here's another fact that grandma may not have known. Drinking two cups of beet juice reduces blood pressure, surprisingly just one to two hours later lasting up to 24 hours, according to a study by British researchers. An article written by Elizabeth Bergman for WebMD Health News, *Nitrates Found in Vegetables May Protect Blood Vessels,* tells us it is the high nitrates in beets which are thought to reduce the blood pressure. Full study results can be found in the February 4, 2008 online edition of *Hypertension*.

Bell Peppers

There's evidence of pepper seed as far back as 5000 BC. It's believed that Spanish and Portuguese explorers carried the seeds throughout South America. Bell peppers are full of vitamins C and A. Free radicals are no match for the carotenoids found in peppers. Red bells, like tomatoes, contain lycopene which studies suggest helps reduce the risk of cervical, bladder, and pancreas cancer. Studies also reveal eating peppers can help with lung disorders, diseases associated with pain, like arthritis, and may help reduce the risk of cataracts. A cup of peppers has only 24 calories.

The fantastic colors of bell peppers add a delicious crunch to lunch buddy salads and wraps. Bells can be roasted, steamed, eaten raw with dips, baked, and stuffed. You'll want to try our Barley Stuffed Peppers on page 147 and Pepper Salad on page 82.

Blackberries

You may also have heard them called black raspberries. Blackberries are a blend of many tiny fruits called drupes, which cluster together on the stem of the plant. Blackberries provide large amounts of anthocyanocide, a key bioflavonoid, and ellagic acid, which is believed to prevent cancers, including colon, oral, and esophageal. Another big benefit you'll receive from eating blackberries is protection against heart disease and stroke. These little berries also help reduce blood sugar levels, add significant amounts of fiber to our diet, and give us folate, as well as vitamins C and E.

Blueberries

Blueberries are one of the super foods that fight against free radicals that damage our cells and DNA. Studies of the phytonutrient anthocyanin in blueberries have shown promise in fighting risks for ovarian cancer, colon cancer, macular degeneration, and Alzheimer's. The phytonutrient may even improve our ability to learn! They contain some of the same properties as cranberries, which prevent urinary tract infections by interfering with bacteria growth. Like blackberries, blueberries also have ellagic acid, a cancer blocker.

Blueberries were introduced to the U.S. early in the 20th century. A botanist at the USDA did extensive research that led to wide production of blueberries in 1916. They're plentiful in supermarkets and it's quite easy to get them into your diet. They add marvelous color to salads, shakes, and cereals. We like to rinse them and eat them right out of the carton. They're high in vitamin C and manganese, a good source of fiber and vitamin E, and have only 81 calories in a cup.

Broccoli

Please don't turn your nose up until you've actually tried it! If you're not eating broccoli, you are missing out on a world of nutrition. First, it's good for the waistline, containing fiber and only 43 calories in a cup. Next, it contains a mighty phytonutrient called sulforaphane which studies have shown can help reduce the risk of colon, ovarian, bladder, lung, and prostate cancer. It's especially high in vitamins C, K, A, and folate. Broccoli is a crucifer that's good for our immune system because of its beta-carotene, which helps the body absorb calcium and vitamin C (also found in broccoli)! You can also get some Omega 3's by eating broccoli.

Here's yet another example of eating the rainbow. According to John Erdman, professor of Food Science and

Human Nutrition at the University of Illinois, when tomatoes and broccoli are eaten together they become an even more powerful team in the fight against prostate cancer. Broccoli even has properties that call into play some enzymes that work at cleansing and detoxifying our bodies.

Ancient Romans ate an early variety of broccoli they called a wild cabbage. Italian immigrants brought broccoli with them when they settled with the colonists in New England and the rest as they say is history!

Cabbage

The smell of cabbage cooking takes Susan back to her great-grandma's kitchen. It's such a versatile vegetable. You can add it to soups, make salads and slaws, steam it, or fry it! If you think you don't like cabbage, start out with some Napa cabbage. Napa cabbage eats like a lettuce with a very, very mild cabbage flavor. Cabbage is in the same crucifer family with broccoli, kale, and Brussels sprouts.

An excellent source of vitamins K and C, cabbage was grown in ancient civilizations and was used to treat many health problems. Its phytonutrients work to lower the risk of cancer more than any other vegetable or fruit.

Organically grown cabbage has a higher level of phytos, and red cabbage has more than the white.

One study of Polish women who had lots of cabbage in their diet found that their rate of breast cancer tripled after they left Poland and began living in the U.S. When cabbage is cut it begins to lose vitamin C, so avoid buying half heads in the supermarket and use it as soon as you cut it.

You'll love our Healing Cabbage Soup on page 215. Aside from the benefits already mentioned, there are only 33 tiny calories in a cup.

Cantaloupe

When you cut into a cantaloupe, it's easy to see by the seeds that it's related to cucumbers and pumpkins. Just one cup of cantaloupe gives you well over your daily allowance of vitamins C and A, with only 56 calories! Vitamin A is a very good nutrient for vision. Eating cantaloupe may even help reduce the risk of getting cataracts and macular degeneration. Smokers would do well to eat foods rich in vitamin A because the cigarette smoke itself causes deficiencies in vitamin A. Studies have shown a lower instance of emphysema in those smokers who ate more vitamin A rich foods.

While the origin of cantaloupes is a bit sketchy, the ancient Greeks and Romans certainly ate them. The colonists were introduced to cantaloupes in early New England.

Choosing a cantaloupe at the supermarket can be a bit daunting, but use your senses. You should smell that sweet perfume but it shouldn't be too strong. Steer away from any melon with dents or soft spots and try giving it a slap with your palm. If it sounds hollow it's probably ripe. Studies have shown that the riper a fruit is, the higher the antioxidants. You can leave a cantaloupe on your counter for a few days to ripen ... just make sure to refrigerate it immediately after cut. Although they're best in the summer, you can also buy some pretty good ones in the winter months.

Carrots

Did you know that thousands of years ago carrots were actually purple? Cultivation over the centuries helped them to become the color we know them today. Researchers believe that the first carrots probably came from a wild plant in Afghanistan. Carrots are the richest source of carotenoids and an excellent source of vitamin A. Did you ever hear that carrots were good for your eyes? Here's why.

Vitamin A travels to the liver then to the retina where it becomes rhodopsin. Rhodopsin is a purple pigment that we need for night vision. Since they are naturally full of antioxidants they can help reduce the risks of some cancers and help regulate blood sugar levels. They're also rich in dietary fiber and minerals, and a cup has about 52 calories. We grate them and slice them into our salads and almost always add them to our soups and stews.

Cauliflower

Cauliflower has a lot of the same cancer fighting substances as broccoli because it's in the same crucifer family. It just lacks the green color because its leaves shade it from the sun, and therefore no chlorophyll is formed. It's an excellent source of vitamins C and K, as well as folate and fiber. Eat cauliflower raw or steamed, and buy organic whenever possible to get the highest level of phytonutrients. Cauliflower contains sulforaphane which, when eaten, signals those detox enzymes to clear out the free radicals. Studies have shown that cauliflower helps reduce the risk of colon, bladder, and lung cancer. In addition, its high amount of vitamin C helps to fight inflammatory diseases such as rheumatoid arthritis. One cup has only 28 calories.

Celery

Celery always reminds us of Thanksgiving and stuffing. We love the smell of it and its delicate flavor. Susan chops a little celery in lots of foods. It's a perfect way for her to get some vegetables into her husband. It's a terrific source of vitamin C, which helps boost our immune system. In addition, it's a natural at lowering blood pressure due to a substance called phalides, which relaxes the muscles around the arteries, thereby promoting cardiovascular health. The high level of vitamin C makes it also very useful in combating inflammatory diseases, such as arthritis and asthma.

Cucumbers

Since the peel of cucumbers is full of fiber and water, what an easy way to get both! Cucumbers give you some vitamin C, and they add a wonderful crunch to salads. Grown in Asia over 10,000 years ago, cucumbers were carried by explorers to other parts of the world. King Louis enjoyed them, and the early colonists brought them to the

United States. Ancient Greeks and Romans used them for skin medicines. Even today they're thought to aid against puffiness around the eyes. Like most vegetables, they're low in calories – just 13 in a whole cup!

Eggplant

Eggplants are the pretty, deep purple vegetable that grows on vines like their cousin, the tomato. They're also related to the sweet pepper and potato. Eggplants were first eaten as they grew wild in India and were cultivated as early as the 5th century BC in China. Thanks to the explorers, they made their way to Italy and finally throughout the world.

The early varieties of eggplant were so bitter they were planted mainly for ornamentation in gardens. At the time, it was believed that eggplant caused insanity and cancer.

The skin contains an anthocyanin phytonutrient called nasunin, which is a potent antioxidant and free radical scavenger protecting our cells from damage. In animal studies, nasunin shows promise in protecting cell membranes in the brain. Eggplant also contains chlorogenic acid, which is one of the most potent free radical scavengers found in plant tissues, giving it enormous anti-cancer and anti-viral properties.

Eggplant can be roasted, steamed, and fried. The peel can be consumed if it isn't too tough, or you can peel it before cooking. To help remove some of the bitterness, salt the flesh and let it sit for about half an hour. This will pull out some of the water, too. Rinse the salt off, and cook as you desire. Eggplant is a good source of fiber, manganese, copper, potassium, and B vitamins such as B1, B6, and B3. Eggplant contains only a wee 27 or so calories in a cup.

Fennel

Susan didn't quite know what to do with her first purchase of fennel. She cut and discarded everything except the stalks and chopped them into our salad. Later she learned you can eat all of it! It's a really gorgeous vegetable which has a bulb, stalks like celery, and fronds like dill. But it doesn't taste like celery or dill. If you haven't tried it yet, please do! Try to plan your lunch buddy meals around it, utilizing all of it in different recipes. You'll need to use it within a week to get the maximum flavor from it.

Use the bulb in your salad to add crunch, and use the stalks and fronds chopped into soups or other dishes.

Keep in mind that your local supermarket may call it anise. It took Susan and the clerk a very long time to figure out how to ring it up. Looking at their list of produce, Susan remembered it's sometimes called anise because of its very mild licorice taste. Count on fennel to deliver an excellent dose of vitamin C and fiber. It's also a good source of potassium, manganese, phosphorus, calcium, magnesium, and vitamin B. There are only 26 calories to a cup. Give it a try in our Spinach Fennel Salad with Oranges on page 85.

Garlic

Garlic has been around for over 6,000 years. It's been worshipped, used in place of antibiotics, and even used for money. Americans didn't catch on to garlic until the 1940's and now it's being worshipped once again! Today we see its value in cardiovascular health. It has some blood thinning properties, can slow the growth of tumors, and helps reduce LDL, the lousy cholesterol. When garlic is cut, chopped, or pressed, there's a sulfur molecule that's changed and we absorb it through our lungs and into our bloodstream. And I think we all know how it escapes … through our breath! But garlic can sweeten as it cooks too.

Just try our South of the Border Garlic Soup on page 182 and get your breath on!

Grapes

Ah, the little grape! A thoroughly portable little food they're great for snacking. But I bet you didn't know that they contain over 600 phytonutrients with antioxidant properties! With only 61 calories per cup, they contain a couple of flavonoids. Flavonoids give foods their color; the deeper the color the higher the flavonoids. Quercitin, one of the flavonoids in grapes, is in a category called resveratrol. Now what does all this mean? Many studies have been done with this compound and the results are staggering! Resveratrol can lower the risks of Alzheimer's, colorectal cancer, and lung diseases. It is also heart protective and can improve blood flow to the brain, thus reducing the risk for stroke!

Researchers who've studied the French diet with its high consumption of fats have shown that the French have a lower rate of heart attacks, which could be as a result of eating grapes and drinking wine. Adding three glasses of dark red wine (the highest in resveratrol) to a meal just three times a week can give you these boosts in health. If you don't drink alcohol, you can still take advantage of the benefits by drinking Concord grape juice . . . but you'll have to drink 25 glasses of juice weekly.

Grapefruit

While high in vitamin C, grapefruits are low in calories. They were first brought to attention in the 18th century, and are thought to be a cross of two fruits, the orange and the pomelo. They received their name by the way they grow in clusters, just like grapes.

Again, the riper the fruit the more antioxidants it offers. Vitamin C has been shown in studies to help reduce the risks of the common cold. But grapefruits give us so much more. They guard against arthritis, heart disease, stroke, and cancers. Grapefruits contain phytonutrients called limonoids. Limonoids slow tumor growth. The pink and red ones contain lycopene, a carotenoid phytonutrient that battles free radicals.

Many studies have been conducted into the benefits of grapefruit juice. If you're prone to kidney stones, drinking grapefruit juice reduces your risk. The juice helps the liver detoxify and aids in the reduction of triglycerides.

The flavonoid naringenin, found in grapefruits, is thought to be able to repair damaged DNA in prostate cancer.

Kale

Crunchy, curly, kale is another one of those foods that, while packed with nutrition, is very low in calories. Furthermore, it's in the family of cabbage that has those detoxifying enzymes called into play when it is chewed or chopped. Kale is an outstanding source of vitamins A, C, and K, and a good source of fiber, calcium, and manganese.

It's believed that early Celtics brought kale to Europe about 600 BC. Ancient Romans and peasants ate kale, and it found its way to the U.S. by way of English settlers.

We chop kale into our salads, but it can also be steamed or added to soups. Be sure to wash the leaves very well to remove dirt and grit.

Kiwifruit

Did you ever wonder why you didn't see this lovely green fruit when you were growing up? That's because it wasn't available in the U.S. until the 1960's. A produce importer brought Kiwi over from New Zealand. She named it kiwifruit after a New Zealand bird that's brown and fuzzy called a kiwi. But kiwi has its roots in China and was originally called Yang Tao. It's a powerhouse of vitamin C, and is a good source of fiber and potassium. We peel and slice our kiwi, but you can rub the fuzz off and eat the peel too, which will give you more fiber. If you're adding it to a salad, put it in right before eating because, like bananas, kiwifruit can become mushy.

Leeks

The ancient ruler Nero ate leeks often because he believed they made his voice stronger and clearer. Leeks are in the onion family and, in fact, look like really big scallions. So they have the same properties as onions, only in smaller amounts and a less strong odor and flavor. Leeks were brought to Wales and the Welsh, who used them during a fight with the Saxons way back in 1620, revered them. The Welsh soldiers put leeks in their hats so they would stand out from the enemy, and then successfully won the battle against the Saxons.

Store them unwashed and when you're ready to use them wash them carefully, separating the green leaves to remove any dirt and grit. And the next time you have a fight with your husband or other male, you might want to stick a leek in your hat. You just might win! If nothing else, you'll get a good laugh from the look on his face when he sees you with a leek in your hat.

Lemons and Limes

Adding fresh lemon and lime juice to food provides a clean, fresh taste and aroma! Make sure to choose lemons that are very yellow and limes that are very green. Be sure to wash them well before using to remove any wax and pesticides, or simply buy organic!

The Crusaders and Christopher Columbus are responsible for carrying the seeds and trees to California and Florida. Lemons and limes didn't grow well in California, and during the gold rush the forty-niners were willing to pay as much as a dollar apiece for them. Why? Because their high concentration of vitamin C prevented scurvy!

Lemons and limes have flavonoids called limonoids, which help prevent cancers of the skin, mouth, stomach, breast, and lung by inhibiting tumor growth. Well worth a buck, aren't they?

Mango

Mangos have natural sugars and are an excellent source of beta-carotene, vitamins C, A, and E, niacin,

Raw Foods Fit for Royalty

potassium, iron, and dietary fiber. Mangos were introduced to California in the 1800's, and are rapidly gaining popularity. We add them to our salads for a juicy sweetness. They're a bit difficult to prepare. Cut slices from each side and scoop out the flesh or peel and slice.

While visiting her cousin Steve in Texas, Susan ate at an authentic Mexican Restaurant. She loved the salsa there so much that the next evening Steve made tomato and mango salsa, his favorite. (See recipes on page 235). He was right about the mango salsa! Back at home Susan brought both to work (for a food day, of course) and the mango salsa disappeared long before the tomato salsa! Try his recipes and see which one you like best.

Onions

If you are eating at Susan's house, you need to tell her if you don't like onions. She puts them in almost everything! She started eating green onions from her grandma's garden, but she especially likes the taste of red onions in salads. The onions she uses the most in everyday cooking are the yellow ones. Guess what? The yellow ones have the most flavonoids!

A cousin of garlic, they're high in vitamin C and quercitin. Because they're high in chromium they can help reduce blood sugar levels. But eating onions can also reduce risks for many diseases. Are you ready? Simply by eating onions, you will reduce your risk of colon cancer, oral cancer, esophageal cancer, larynx cancer, breast and ovarian cancer, prostate cancer, and renal (kidney) cancer. And that's not all! Women who suffer from osteoporosis or osteopeania, as Susan and I do, can benefit from eating onions. Researchers have recently found that onions guard against osteoclasts. MedicineNet.com defines an osteoclast as "a cell that nibbles at and breaks down bone, responsible for bone resorption."

Remember the Israelites who missed onions? They were paid with onions in return for their hard work on the pyramids! Onions were highly prized by the Egyptians. The Ancient Egyptians even put onions in the tombs of their kings to be carried with them into the afterlife. It's believed that Columbus took them to the West Indies, and their popularity grew from there.

Oranges

Don't you just love it when someone is peeling an orange? The aroma seems to fill the room. Did you know they are one of the most popular fruits? We know oranges are loaded with vitamin C, but they're also a good source of dietary fiber. Among other benefits, oranges may protect against many cancers, arthritis, ulcers, kidney stones, and strokes. Their phytonutrients are called citrus flavanones. Oranges can also help lower blood pressure and cholesterol. We like to add orange sections to our salads. One of our favorite salads is simply baby spinach leaves and orange sections. All you need is a light vinaigrette and a sprinkle of walnuts to complement this very nutritious salad. Yum!

Papaya

We have to admit our first exposure to papaya wasn't good! Susan didn't know how to select one. But that won't be true for you. Pick papayas that are a red orange color. They should be soft, but not too soft. Black spots on them won't hurt. If they're yellow, they'll need a few more days to ripen. If they're green, don't buy them at all. To prepare them, wash and cut in half lengthwise. Then scoop out the seeds. Their sweet velvety flesh can be eaten like a melon with a spoon or use a melon baller. Papayas are a great source of vitamins C, A, E, and K, folate, potassium, and fiber. They contain carotenes that are good for cardiovascular health, and may guard against colon cancer and macular degeneration.

Pears

We like pears when they're very ripe, when they seem to almost melt in your mouth. They're usually still hard when we buy them. When we put them in the bottom of our fruit bowl with apples and bananas, they soon ripen. The riper they are, the more antioxidants you get! Did you know pears are a member of the rose family and a cousin to apples? Historians speculate that pears were first around in the Stone Age! They're a good source of vitamin C, fiber, and copper. Copper helps protect us from free radicals and, of course, our bodies love the cholesterol reducing fiber. Try our Romaine, Pear, and Walnut Salad on page 84!

Pineapples

Discovered in the late 1400's by explorers, it became clear that a tropical climate was needed for this fruit to flourish. Did you know a pineapple is not just one fruit, but is a composite of many flowers whose individual fruitlets are bound to a central core? One cup of pineapple can give you over 100% of the trace mineral manganese. Pineapple is also rich in vitamin B1. Both manganese and vitamin B1 give us energy. Pineapple also helps with digestion. Here again, the more ripe the fruit the more antioxidant activity. Pineapple is a good source of copper, fiber, and B6. It's fabulous in our Lunch Buddy Fruit Salad on page 77 and has just 75 calories in a cup.

Plums

Plums are very portable and easy to pack in your lunch. Just remember to eat them when they're very ripe to get the maximum flavor and benefits. Put them in your fruit bowl for a few days when you bring them home from the store so that they ripen fully.

They give us a good dose of vitamins C, A, and B2, as well as fiber and potassium. Plums contain phytonutrients called phenols. These phenols can help prevent oxidation to fats in our brain and in our blood. Related to peaches, they're called a drupe, a fruit that surrounds itself around a pit. Plums have been consumed for over 2,000 years ... and the Pilgrims are responsible for bringing them to the U.S. in the 17th century. There are over a thousand varieties of plums but the ones we are most familiar with range in color from red to a deep purple, almost black. The sweet inside flesh can be yellowish, pink, or red.

Raisins

Ancient civilizations consumed raisins over 2,000 years ago, and raisins are even mentioned in the Bible. Romans often used them for money and awarded them to winners of competitions. Today the largest producer of raisins is located in the San Joaquin Valley in California. Back in the late 1800's an extremely hot season ruined the grapes in this region, or so it seemed. A grower took the dried grapes to market and the rest is history.

Raisins give us an important source of boron. Boron is particularly helpful in aiding bone health and possesses some of the advantages of estrogen, making raisins a great food choice for menopausal women. Raisins are very sweet, and while they have fewer amounts of phenols as compared to grapes, they are still full of antioxidants. A quarter of a cup has about 108 calories.

Radicchio

Radicchio has Italian roots and is a member of the chicory family. It's so pretty with its scarlet color. Including radicchio in your salad adds magnesium, potassium, and vitamin A, as well as color and crunch.

Raspberries

These delectable red delicate berries have been with us since prehistoric times and most likely originated in Asia. Related to the rose, these bramble-growing yummies are big in nutrition and friendly to the waistline. One cup of raspberries is only about 60 calories. You'll see them more plentiful from early summer to early fall. Wash them carefully to avoid injuring them. If you see any spoiled or moldy ones, pick those out to avoid contamination of the other berries. Make sure you eat them in a day or two. Raspberries are high in manganese, antioxidants, vitamin C, and fiber. Like blueberries and blackberries, they also have ellagic acid.

Romaine Lettuce

Romaine lettuce is very low in calories (2 cups contain only 15 calories), and it's a very nutritious addition to your meal. It contains many nutrients that contribute to a heart-healthy diet, including folate, potassium, and vitamins A and C. Romaine is a good source of dietary fiber, chromium, and manganese. Beta-carotene and vitamin C work to reduce cholesterol and you get both of these in romaine. Experts believe that romaine dates as far back as 4500 BC. Ancient Romans and Greeks used it for medicines, and the Chinese still serve it on special days for good luck. When choosing a lettuce for salads or sandwiches, skip the iceberg and go for the romaine.

Spinach

Canned spinach is the main reason people say they don't like spinach. Let's face it, the slimy green mess that slides out of a can just doesn't look appetizing! It wasn't until a few years ago that we actually ate raw spinach. What a difference!

Just recently, while putting a package of it on the checkout counter at the supermarket, Susan's husband remarked that he was glad that he didn't have to eat that stuff. She had to laugh because she had been chopping it in his salads for quite a while!

Do you want to know the reason that spinach is called a super food? How about a bunch of reasons?

Spinach has at least three flavonoids that function as antioxidants. It's so nutrient-packed that it can help protect against colon cancer, osteoporosis, heart disease, arthritis, and ovarian and prostate cancer. Not only that, it's good for your brain and even for your eyesight! It's rich in vitamins K, C, B2, and B6, as well as folate, magnesium, manganese, iron, calcium, fiber, and copper. It also contains omega 3's and of course it's very low in calories.

Spinach is in the same family with Swiss chard and beets. When you bring it home, don't wash it. Just roll it gently in paper toweling and put it all in a plastic storage bag. It can last up to two weeks this way.

Wash it only as you need it. If you long ago (in the days of Popeye) turned your mind against spinach, come back! Try it sautéed in olive oil (don't tell Popeye), or raw in salads. We think you'll be a fan.

Summer Squash

The most popular varieties of summer squash are zucchini, yellow squash, and pattypan squash. The first squash, eaten over 10,000 years ago, was seedy, bitter, and didn't contain much flesh. Christopher Columbus brought squash to Europe, and other explorers were responsible for introducing them in other areas of the world.

Related to melons and cucumbers, they are an excellent source of manganese. Other nutrients found in squash are vitamins C, K, and B6, as well as magnesium, copper, folate, phosphorus, iron, and protein. Squash even contains some omega 3 fatty acids, which help reduce risks for heart attack, stroke, and atherosclerosis.

Enjoy them roasted, cooked, or raw in salads. We like them roasted with barley or couscous.

Sweet Potatoes

Is it a yam or is it a sweet potato? Well, sweet potatoes have many different names across the world, but the ones we eat today get their name from an African word for describing the root of the plant. When they were introduced to the U.S., they were given the name yam to separate them from a common sweet white potato. The orange-fleshed ones we are familiar with are really sweet potatoes. To add to the confusion, the Department of Agriculture requires yams to also be labeled as sweet potatoes.

There should be no confusion though about all of the benefits they can give us. Sweet potatoes are an excellent source of vitamins A and C, and a good source of fiber, potassium, copper, iron, and vitamin B6. Sweet potatoes are heart healthy and can help reduce the symptoms of arthritis and asthma. Studies have also shown them to guard against colon cancer. While prehistoric populations ate sweet potatoes, explorers are responsible for scattering them throughout the world.

Swiss Chard

This lovely green isn't native to Switzerland, but got its name from a Swiss botanist in the 19th century who named it after his homeland. Swiss Chard originally hails from the Mediterranean. It's easy to see that it is related to beets by the pretty red stem running through the very large and wrinkly leaves. Other close cousins are mustard, turnip greens, and spinach. You'll want to wash the leaves very well just before using to get rid of the sandy grit. We like it cut up in our green salads and have used it in soups and pasta dishes. We also like it steamed with hot sauce. In addition, the leaves are large enough to use for a wrap instead of a tortilla.

It is a truly fabulous super food! Just by eating one serving of Swiss chard, you will take in over 700% of your daily requirement of vitamin K and over 100% of vitamin A, important for vision health. It's an excellent source of vitamin C, magnesium, and manganese. But that's not all. It gives us iron for energy, fiber, zinc, copper, folate, phosphorus, potassium, vitamin E, protein, calcium, and vitamin B2! Swiss chard is heart healthy and can help reduce risks for certain cancers, as well as emphysema. As we age our mental sharpness may decline but studies have shown that eating three servings of green leafy or yellow cruciferous veggies daily can actually slow down this decline.

Tomatoes

The benefits of tomatoes are simply staggering. They deliver high amounts of vitamins C, A, and K, and the carotenoid, lycopene. Studies suggest that tomatoes are heart-healthy and cancer-preventing. Tomato juice may help reduce blood clots and is a natural anti-inflammatory. We have tomatoes in our soups and salads, and we also have a glass of low sodium V-8 almost every day.

Watermelon

Mmmmmm! Watermelon is a delightfully sweet and refreshing treat that actually quenches your thirst. Even though it tastes as sweet as candy, it only has 48 calories in a cup. Since it has very high water content and is low in calories, it delivers more nutrients per ounce than many other fruits. Watermelon delivers a big punch of vitamins A, C, B6, and B1. It can help reduce some symptoms of asthma, diabetes, colon cancer, arthritis, and atherosclerosis. The B vitamins in watermelon are required for energy production in our bodies. Watermelon contains the powerful beta-carotene, lycopene, that tracks down those pesky damaging free radicals and is believed to reduce the risk of prostate cancer.

A native of Africa, watermelon was first grown for food in Egypt. Drawings of watermelons on the inside walls of the tombs of Egyptian kings prove that they often went into the afterlife with this wonderful fruit as a companion. Ancient people enjoyed watermelon as food and as water in times of drought.

So if you are thinking of cutting out sugary desserts, go ahead and have some watermelon instead!

Balsamic Strawberry Salad

- ¼ cup balsamic vinaigrette (see recipe below)
- ½ pint fresh strawberries, hulled and thinly sliced
- 1 tablespoon balsamic vinegar
- 5 ounces organic Baby Arugula
- ½ cup pecan halves, toasted
- Kosher salt and freshly ground pepper to taste

Prepare Balsamic Vinaigrette by adding 4 tablespoons extra virgin olive oil to 2 tablespoons of balsamic vinegar. Add kosher salt and freshly ground pepper to taste.

To toast pecan halves or other nuts and seeds, preheat oven to 350°, and spread nuts in a shallow baking pan. Bake 5 to 10 minutes or till light golden brown. Stir once or twice so they don't burn, and keep an eye on them. Toasting enhances the flavor of nuts and seeds.

Toss the strawberries with one tablespoon balsamic vinegar. Marinate for 10 minutes.

Add the Baby Arugula and pecan halves to the marinated strawberries. Add vinaigrette to taste and gently toss. Season with salt and pepper to taste, and serve immediately.

<u>**Lunch Buddy Notes**</u> – Arugula is an excellent source of folate, vitamins A and C, and provides over 100% of your daily vitamin K. In addition, it is a good source of calcium, magnesium, and manganese, making it a superfood for your bones.

Recipe adapted from Jennifer Chandler's book, <u>Simply Salads</u>. She has created more than 100 recipes using prepackaged greens. These salads couldn't be easier, or more delicious. You'll want to pick up this book to add to your collection. This is one of our favorites.

Makes 6 servings.

Black Bean and Wild Rice Salad

- 1 6-ounce box wild rice
- 14 ounces vegetable broth
- 1 bay leaf
- 1 can black beans, drained and rinsed
- ½ green or red bell pepper, chopped
- 1 14.5 ounce can diced tomatoes with juice
- ½ bunch green onions, chopped
- 1 clove garlic, chopped

Dressing

- ½ cup extra virgin olive oil
- ¼ cup orange juice
- 1 tablespoon chili powder
- 1 tablespoon cumin
- ¼ cup chopped cilantro (about ¼ of a bunch)

Prepare rice according to the package using the broth in place of the water. Add bay leaf. When the rice is done, remove the bay leaf and add the other ingredients. Pour dressing over all and toss to blend.

Makes 4 to 6 servings.

Black Bean Salsa Salad

- 1 can (about 15 ounces) black beans, drained and rinsed
- ½ small red onion, chopped
- 2 cloves garlic, chopped or minced
- 1 handful of fresh cilantro, chopped
- 2 tomatoes, seeded and chopped
- 2 mangoes, cubed
- 1 orange
- 3 limes

Combine beans, onion, garlic, cilantro, tomatoes, and mangoes in a medium bowl with a lid.

Zest and juice the orange and lime into a small bowl. Whisk together and pour over salad. Serve chilled.

Makes 4 servings.

Citrus/Mango Salad with Toasted Walnuts

- 1 red apple
- 1 green apple
- 1 mango
- 1 orange
- 1 lemon
- Walnuts, toasted (about ½ cup)

Preheat oven to 350°.

Place walnuts in a single layer on a cookie sheet. Bake in the oven 5-7 minutes, until you can smell them.

Dice the apples and mango and place in a bowl that will have a lid. Use a zester to cut long strips of orange and lemon peel, and toss in with the fruit. Juice the orange and lemon into the fruit. Cover and refrigerate, preferably overnight. Serve sprinkled with the toasted walnuts.

<u>**Lunch Buddy Notes**</u> – This would be a very pretty salad served on a lettuce cup or a bed of spinach.

Makes 3 servings.

Cucumber and Carrot Salad

Note: Make the dressing if possible the day before or several hours prior to serving.

- 6 romaine leaves, chopped or torn
- 1 carrot, shredded
- 1 small or ½ large cucumber, sliced into small chunks

Toss all together; add dill dressing to taste.

Dill Dressing

- ¼ cup white wine vinegar
- ¼ teaspoon dried or ¾ teaspoon fresh dill, chopped
- 4 tablespoons extra virgin olive oil

Combine all ingredients.

Makes 4 servings.

Dr. Weil's Citrus Dressing

- ⅓ cup freshly squeezed orange or grapefruit juice
- 2 tablespoons organic balsamic vinegar
- 1 tablespoon extra virgin olive oil
- Salt and black pepper to taste

Whisk all ingredients together and use within 5 days.

<u>**Lunch Buddy Notes**</u> – We usually use an orange, although grapefruit would also be very good. We don't add any salt or pepper because with all the tasty ingredients in our salad, we find it isn't necessary. Sometimes after storing in the refrigerator, the olive oil solidifies a bit. Just take the dressing out of the refrigerator about ½ hour before you are going to use it, and be sure to shake it up.

Gil's Salad

- Celery
- Lettuce
- Tomatoes
- Green Onions
- Radishes
- Cauliflower or broccoli
- Any other vegetable you like
- ¼ to ½ cup grated parmesan cheese
- ¼ cup to ½ cup Italian dressing

Chop vegetables in equal portions. Combine in a large bowl with dressing ingredients. Let sit for about an hour.

<u>*Lunch Buddy Notes*</u> – This recipe was created by the husband of a retired coworker, who doesn't like fruits and vegetables. Her favorite foods are hot dogs and candy. Her husband convinced her to try this salad, and she loves it! Congratulations, Gil! Our recommendation ... try it, you'll love it!

Make as much or as little as you like.

Grapefruit and Avocado Salad

- 1 grapefruit, peeled
- ½ white onion, halved and thinly sliced
- 2 ripe avocados, halved, peeled, and cut into thin slices
- 1 bag (7 ounces) Riviera Blend (or any blend of radicchio and butter lettuce)
- 3 tablespoons extra virgin olive oil
- Kosher salt and freshly ground pepper

Separate the grapefruit slices over a large salad bowl, catching the juice in the bowl. Remove the seeds.

Add the grapefruit slices to the bowl. Add the onion, avocados, Riviera Blend, and olive oil. Gently toss.

Season with salt and pepper to taste.

Lunch Buddy Notes – From Simply Salads, by Jennifer Chandler. To get the juiciest and most colorful grapefruit (or orange) slices for your salads, remove the peel with a sharp knife. Be sure to remove all of the white pith. Then cut between the membranes to separate the segments. Before discarding, squeeze the remaining membranes over the bowl to capture all the luscious juices for your dressing.

Makes 6 servings.

Lentil & Garbanzo Bean Salad

- 1 cup of lentils
- 2 carrots, sliced
- 1 teaspoon cumin seeds
- 1 bay leaf
- 2½ cups water
- ¼ cup fresh basil leaves, chopped
- ¼ cup fresh mint leaves, chopped
- ¼ cup fresh oregano, chopped
- 10 grape or cherry tomatoes, cut in half lengthwise
- 1 small bunch green onions, sliced
- 1 15-ounce can garbanzo beans, drained and rinsed
- 4 tablespoons extra virgin olive oil
- Juice and zest of one lemon
- Kosher or sea salt and ground black pepper

Cook the lentils, carrots, cumin seeds, and bay leaf in the water until the lentils are tender, about 25 minutes. Drain and put into a large bowl to cool.

Add the chopped herbs, tomatoes, green onions, and garbanzo beans. Mix the olive oil, lemon juice, and zest of lemon.

Pour into the lentil salad. Season with salt and pepper to taste. Cover and refrigerate before serving. If you prefer, this is very good heated.

Makes 4 servings.

Lunch Buddy Salad

- Romaine Lettuce
- Bok Choy
- Kale
- Radicchio
- Red or Green Onion
- Celery
- Sweet peppers
- Radishes
- Tomatoes
- Spinach
- Carrot
- Blueberries
- Orange
- Mango
- Walnuts

Chop all of the ingredients except walnuts and put in a bowl. You can add one or all three fruits. Toss together and put into bowls or arrange nicely on a plate. Top with walnuts. You don't need a lot of these ingredients to make a large salad, so make as much or as little as you like. We usually make enough for two days. The vegetables remain fresh and it's a timesaver that second day. Try squeezing a lemon or an orange over the salad, or use our favorite Dr. Andrew Weil salad dressing on page 72.

Make as much or as little as you like.

Lunch Buddy Fruit Salad

- Fresh Pineapple
- Oranges
- Grapes
- Kiwi Fruit
- Strawberries
- Raspberries
- Blackberries
- Blueberries

Cut the top and bottom off the pineapple and then quarter it from top to bottom. Remove the core and chop pineapple. Put in a large bowl. Peel and chop one large or two small oranges, and add to pineapple. Rinse grapes and slice in half lengthwise. Peel and chop two or three kiwi fruit, and add. Rinse a pint of strawberries, and if they are large, cut in half and add to salad. Rinse red raspberries, blackberries, and blueberries and sprinkle on top of the salad.

Lunch Buddy Notes – You won't need any heavy dressings, cool whip, little marshmallows, or sugar with this salad. The natural sweetness of the fruits will delight your taste buds, and just the sight of it will entice you to devour it. You will usually have enough for two to three days. Bananas don't hold up as well as the other fruit, but if you like them you may want to slice one half of a banana on your salad each day before you eat it. If you can't find one of the fruits, substitute another for it or just leave it out altogether. You can't go wrong with this salad. Use your imagination.

Make as much or as little as you like.

Lunch Buddy Pasta Salad

- 4 cups whole wheat penne rigata pasta
- Salt
- ⅛ to ¼ teaspoon red pepper flakes
- 1 clove garlic, chopped
- 2 green onions, chopped
- ½ cup fresh basil leaves, chopped
- ½ cup fresh oregano leaves, chopped
- ½ cup fresh parsley, chopped
- 14.5 ounce can of diced tomatoes with juice
- Juice of a half of a fresh lemon
- 2 tablespoons extra virgin olive oil
- Freshly grated Parmesan cheese

Season pasta water with salt, and cook whole-wheat pasta according to package directions.

Drain pasta and lightly rinse with cold water, then put into large bowl. Add the red pepper flakes, garlic, green onions, basil, oregano, parsley, tomatoes, lemon juice, and olive oil. Stir to combine all of the ingredients. Best when chilled overnight.

Top with freshly grated Parmesan cheese.

Lunch Buddy Notes – We love this recipe because:

- Just ¾ cup provides 7 grams or 20% of your daily requirement of dietary fiber
- Good source of lycopene (higher concentration in cooked tomatoes)
- No cholesterol
- Good way to use your fresh garden herbs
- Filling, yet low in fat
- Short cooking time

Makes 6 to 8 servings.

Melon Salad with Mint and Honey

- ¼ watermelon, cut in medium cubes
- Cantaloupe balls (about ½ cantaloupe)
- Honey Dew melon balls (about ½ of a melon)
- 4 green onions, sliced using white and green parts
- 1 cup of grapes, sliced in half
- ¼ cup fresh mint, chopped

Mix all ingredients lightly in a bowl and serve immediately drizzled with honey.

Makes 6 to 8 servings.

O Baby! Greens

- 2 cups Mesclun greens (assorted young salad leaves)
- 1 cup baby spinach leaves
- Grape tomatoes, sliced in half
- Your favorite vinaigrette

A mustard dressing stands up well to the spicy mesclun. Makes 4 servings.

Vinaigrettes

Mustard Vinaigrette
- 4 tablespoons walnut oil
- 1 tablespoons balsamic vinegar
- 2 teaspoons Dijon mustard
- Touch of sea salt and pepper

Whisk well.

Cumin Vinaigrette (without vinegar)
- Juice and zest of two limes
- 1 teaspoon honey
- 1 teaspoon ground cumin
- 4 tablespoons extra virgin olive oil
- Touch of sea salt and pepper

Whisk and serve, or chill and serve.

Strawberry Vinaigrette
- 6 strawberries, hulled and sliced
- 1 tablespoon red wine vinegar
- 3 tablespoons extra virgin olive oil
- 2 teaspoons honey

Add to a blender and liquefy.

Pepper Salad

- 1 green bell pepper, chopped
- 1 yellow bell pepper, chopped
- 1 red bell pepper, chopped
- 3 medium thick slices of red onion, chopped
- 1 large clove garlic, finely minced (by hand or with a garlic press)
- 3-4 Roma tomatoes, cut into chunks
- 1 large or 2 small cucumbers, sliced
- 3-4 sprigs fresh oregano, pull leaves from stem
- ¼ cup cider or white wine vinegar
- 4 tablespoons extra virgin olive oil
- Sea salt
- Black pepper

Combine all vegetables and fresh oregano leaves in a bowl with a lid. Whisk cider or white wine vinegar, olive oil, sea salt, and pepper until blended. Pour over vegetables and marinate overnight.

Lunch Buddy Notes – This is a great way to enjoy your fresh garden produce.

Makes 4 servings.

Red and Green Salad

- 1 large leaf of Swiss chard, chopped or torn, including red stem
- ½ raw beet, shredded
- ¼ red bell pepper, diced

Toss together with red wine vinaigrette (recipe follows).

Makes 2 servings.

Red Wine Vinaigrette

- ¼ cup red wine vinegar
- 4 tablespoons extra virgin olive oil

Mix together.

<u>Lunch Buddy Notes</u> – Spice up your vinaigrettes with either fresh or dried herbs such as oregano or basil.

Romaine and Pear Salad with Walnuts and Chive Flowers

- Several hearts of romaine, chopped or torn into bite size pieces
- 2 very ripe pears, chopped into bite-size pieces
- 1 cup walnuts
- ¼ cup purple chive flowers, lightly sliced in half
- Freshly grated Parmesan cheese

Serve with your favorite vinaigrette.

<u>**Lunch Buddy Notes**</u> – The chive flowers are a pretty addition to the salad, but Susan and I found out the hard way ... watch out for ants! Ants can actually survive for quite some time submerged in a sink full of water, and for several hours in the refrigerator. When Susan took the lid off our salad, we had ants running all over the table in our break room. It was quite a scramble to take care of the little buggers!

Makes 4 servings.

Spinach Fennel Salad with Oranges

- 2 cups baby spinach leaves, rinsed and dried
- 1 fennel bulb, sliced or chunked
- 2 oranges

You can tear or chop the spinach leaves, or leave them whole. Place them in a bowl with the fennel. Peel and section the oranges and add to the bowl. Dress with an orange vinaigrette, such as Dr. Weil's Citrus Salad Dressing on page 72.

Makes 2 to 3 servings.

Sweet as Dessert Salad

Prepare dressing in advance:

- ½ cup of corn oil
- ½ cup of cider vinegar
- ½ cup of white sugar
- 4 tablespoons of soy sauce

Mix and boil one minute. Let cool in refrigerator before adding to the cabbage mix. Keep dressing in refrigerator for up to two weeks. Can be used on any salad.

Prepare topping in advance:

- 1 package ramen noodles (break up into small bite-size pieces and toss the seasoning packet)
- 2 tablespoons almond slices
- 2 tablespoons sesame seeds
- 2 tablespoons margarine

Melt the margarine, and add the sesame seeds, almonds, and noodles. Brown in oven at 350°, stirring every 10 minutes for 30 minutes.

Cabbage Mix

- 1 head of Napa cabbage, chopped
- 4 - 6 green onions, chopped

Just before serving, combine salad with 1/3 cup of dressing. Top with 4 tablespoons of topping.

Lunch Buddy Notes – This recipe was shared with me by a waitress at a great little café in a furniture store in Kewanee, Illinois. I changed the recipe slightly by reducing the amount of oil and sugar. Sure there's some sugar in the dressing, but if it gets your loved ones eating cabbage (like it did ours) go ahead. We all know a spoonful of sugar makes the medicine go down! Along with slightly less than two tablespoons of sugar, you get the healthy benefit of the cabbage, including fiber and numerous vitamins, and the sliced almonds. To put this small amount of sugar in perspective, there are 11 tablespoons of sugar in every can of pop. So go ahead, have a little sugar with your cabbage! Just skip the pop.

This is one of my favorite salads for dinner parties because you can prepare everything ahead of time, and assemble just before serving. Just toss the cabbage and green onion in a large baggie, cool the dressing in the refrigerator, and keep the topping on the cabinet (hidden from your family, of course). Just before serving, put cabbage mix in small bowls, mixing with a small amount of dressing, and toss on some of the topping. Or you can place all the cabbage in a large salad bowl, mix with dressing, and sprinkle on the topping.

Even salad haters love this salad!

Makes 6 to 8 servings.

Strawberry Spinach Salad

- 10 ounces fresh spinach
- 2 cups sliced strawberries
- ½ cup thinly sliced red onion (1/2 small)
- ⅓ cup fresh lemon juice (2 lemons)
- 3 tablespoons sugar
- 1 tablespoon canola oil
- 2 teaspoons grated lemon rind
- Freshly ground black pepper
- Sliced almonds

Add sliced strawberries to spinach in a medium bowl. Cut thinly sliced onion into bite-size pieces, and add to strawberries and spinach. Place cover on bowl and refrigerate.

First grate or zest lemon rind. Then juice lemons to make 1/3 cup. Add sugar and oil to lemon zest and juice. Refrigerate. Just before eating, add almonds and lemon vinaigrette to spinach salad, and toss. Serve immediately.

<u>Lunch Buddy Notes</u> – This recipe provides 3.1 grams fiber, 1.6 mg iron, and 58 mg calcium. If you wait to put the dressing on each serving right before you eat it, you can also have it the next day. Otherwise the strawberries break down.

Makes 6 servings.

Tomato Cucumber Salad

- 4 chopped tomatoes
- 2 chopped cucumbers
- ½ cup chopped onions
- 2 minced garlic cloves
- ¼ cup olive oil
- ⅛ cup apple cider vinegar
- 1 teaspoon oregano
- 1 teaspoon basil
- Slivered almonds

Toss all ingredients in a large bowl and marinate one hour. Sprinkle almonds on top when ready to eat.

Lunch Buddy Notes – Great salad for the summer. If using fresh herbs, use 1 tablespoon of each. Can be saved and eaten the second day as long as you sprinkle the almonds on each serving rather than over the entire salad.

Makes 4 servings.

Triple Berry Salad

- 1 pint red raspberries
- 1 pint blackberries
- 1 pint blueberries

Mix in a bowl, and enjoy each bite of this nutritional powerhouse.

<u>*Lunch Buddy Notes*</u> – Berries are a powerhouse of good nutrition and fiber. Nothing could be easier than this fruit salad (or more delicious). If you can't find one of these berries, substitute strawberries or any other fruit of your choice.

Makes 4 servings.

Nuts

Give your health a rocket boost by including a colorful variety of these fruits and vegetables in your salads, and don't forget to toss in about a quarter cup of nuts daily. Adding nuts to your diet could add up to four years to your life, according to a recent news story. Peanuts, walnuts, and almonds are a good source of heart-healthy fat – the kind that increases your good cholesterol and decreases your bad.

<u>Lunch Buddy Notes</u> – Toasting enhances the flavor of nuts and seeds. To toast, preheat oven to 350°, and spread in a shallow pan. Bake 5 to 10 minutes or till light golden brown. Stir once or twice so they don't burn, and keep an eye on them.

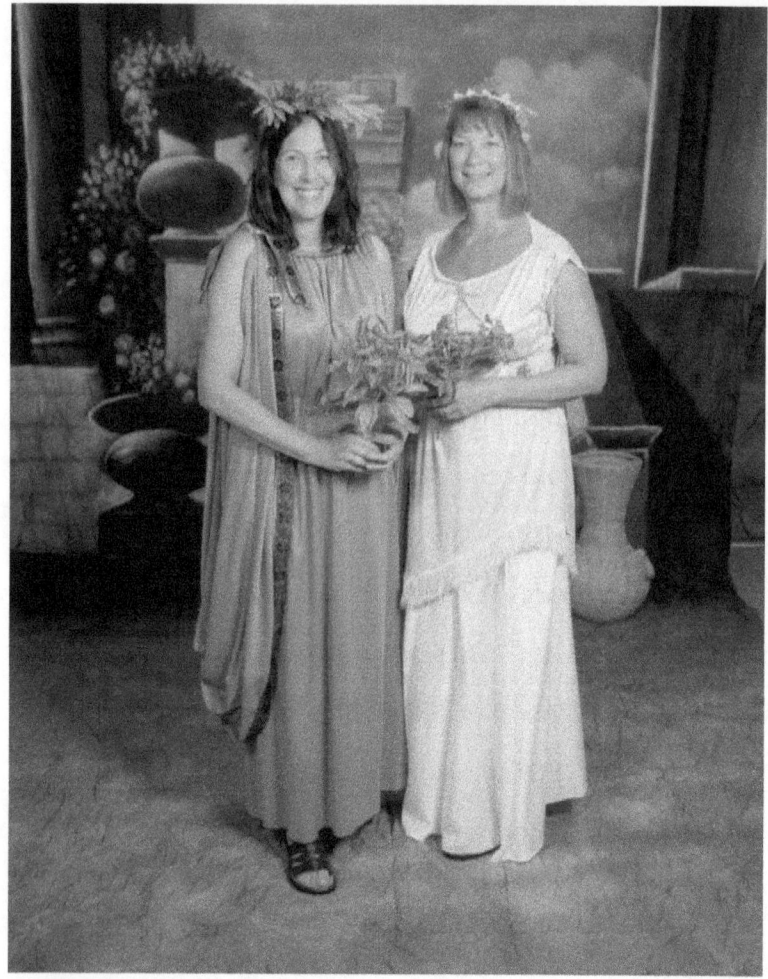

Photo 3 – At least 52 herbs are woven into the tales of Greek mythology.

Heavenly Herbs and Spices

Throughout history herbs have been used as medicines, colognes, foods, seasonings, disinfectants, and even as currency. In the earliest cultures, herbal use was intertwined with spiritualism, mythology, magic, and ritualism. Evidence of the use of herbs can be traced back to a 60,000-year-old burial site in Iraq, which contained eight different medicinal plants, most likely intended to be taken along in the afterlife.

While herbs are mentioned in the Bible, more than 52 herbs and plants are mentioned in the tales of Greek mythology, an ancient religion practiced more than 5,000 years ago. Here are a few of these tales.

Zeus, the main god of the ancient Greeks, became enraged at his cousin, Prometheus, and took fire from man to punish him. Prometheus gave the fire back to man in a hollow fennel stem.

Most of us remember Cupid and his arrows, but may not have ever heard the whole story. Apollo was teasing Cupid about his tiny arrows. Interesting ... it appears that men have been teasing each other about the size of their tools for centuries. Yep, you know what I'm thinking about, don't you? To get back at Apollo, Cupid shot an arrow of love into Apollo's heart. He then turned to a nymph standing nearby, Daphne, and shot an arrow to repel into her heart. Apollo fell deeply in love with her, and began to chase her. She ran away from him, but he was too fast. When he started to catch her, she called out to her father to save her. Her father turned her into a Laurus nobilis (bay laurel) tree. Apollo grabbed the tree and cried out, "My love, my love, I shall love you forever and evermore you shall be green. I will wear your leaves as a crown to remember you." Even today bay wreaths are used as a sign of victory and honor to poets and conquerors.

Want to hear a story which could have been the basis for the world's first soap opera? Mentha was a beautiful nymph who fell in love with Pluto. His wife, Persephone, after learning of Mentha's love for Pluto, turned her into a mint plant. The botanical name for spearmint is Mentha viridis and peppermint is Mentha piperita.

While many Greeks believed that scorpions would breed under pots of basil, in India basil was considered a sacred herb, one which if buried with them would be their passport to heaven. The ancient Romans believed that eating basil would protect them against Basilisk, the fire breathing dragon, and some people even today believe that if you put some basil in your wallet, you will be rich and successful. Anybody want to try it and let us know if it works?

Parsley was considered the herb of the dead. It was said to have sprung up from the blood of the Greek hero Archemorus, the forerunner of death. The ancient Greeks dedicated this herb to Persephone, goddess of the underworld, and used it in funeral rites.

The ancient Greek, Roman, Celtic, Arabic, and Chinese cultures, in fact every early culture on earth, relied upon the therapeutic qualities of herbs and other plants for healing. From Hippocrates (468 – 377 BC) in Greece, to Claudius Galenus (AD 131 – 199) in Rome, to the Yellow Emperor in China (reputed to have lived around 2500 BC), the basis for their medicine was to use herbs and plants to treat the disharmonies (diseases) of the time, believed to have been caused by a lack of balance in the elements making up each person.

Hippocrates, known today as the father of medicine, placed all foods and herbs into categories, based upon their qualities – hot, cold, dry, or damp. He believed that good health was a result of keeping these qualities in balance, as well as exercising and breathing in fresh air.

Galen, utilizing many of the old Hippocratic ideas, wrote a book which soon became the standard medical text for Romans, and for later Arab and medieval physicians. His theories are still an integral part of Unani medicine today.

Like Hippocrates, the Yellow Emperor and the ancient Chinese saw illness as a sign of disharmony within the person, and based their medicine on a theory of elements. The Chinese theory of opposites, *yin and yang*, complemented the theory of elements. The theory of opposites described *yin* as female, dark and cold, while *yang* was described as male, light and hot. Even today, in traditional Chinese medicine, it is believed that *yin and yang* need to be in balance in order to maintain good health.

These stories merely scratch the surface of the history of herbs. If you are interested in learning more, <u>The</u>

Heavenly Herbs and Spices

Complete Medicinal Herbal, by Penelope Ody is an excellent resource.

Surprisingly, some of the herbal remedies used in ancient days are utilized even today. Hemp, used for eye problems in the days of Rameses III, is sometimes prescribed for glaucoma today. Garlic, used medicinally for at least 5,000 years, is known today for its ability to reduce cholesterol levels, for reducing the risk of subsequent heart attacks in cardiac patients, and as a stimulant for the immune system.

In his book, 8 Weeks to Optimum Health, Dr. Andrew Weil says, "Garlic is a superior tonic for the cardiovascular system" and goes on to describe its very important cardiovascular effects. It lowers blood pressure, cholesterol, and triglycerides, while inhibiting blood clotting by reducing the tendency of platelets to clump together. He also tells us that epidemiologists believe that the high consumption of garlic in parts of Spain and Italy may have contributed to a lower than expected incidence of coronary heart disease in those areas. Worried about your breath? Dr. Weil says, "If you eat garlic regularly, any odor from it should hardly be noticeable." And if your family and friends eat it too (as they should), who's going to notice?

Dr. William Withering, who published his *Acccount of the Foxglove and Some of Its Medical Uses* in 1785, spent 10 years studying the side effects of foxglove. He astutely realized that great care was needed in its administration, as the therapeutic dose is very close to the quantity causing toxic side effects. After further analysis, the cardiac glycosides digoxin and digitoxin were eventually extracted. The common foxglove is still used to produce digitoxin, which is currently in use for treating heart conditions today.

Many people today are turning to holistic and herbal medicine in an effort to avoid some of the not-so-favorable consequences of traditional medicine. We are certainly not experts on this topic, but we do believe through a better diet including herbal enhancements we can avoid many of the diseases and conditions so prevalent today. That said we also believe in the value of traditional medicine.

Susan's first serious experience with fresh herbs was when she bought a small basil plant from her friend Sandy who had a stand of fresh herbs at a farmer's market. She

Heavenly Herbs and Spices

planted the basil in big wooden planter and it grew into a large bush. Sandy introduced her to basil pesto and different ways to use it, and now Susan plants no fewer than three basil plants every spring. This summer Susan was really pleased to give some basil back to Sandy – a large plastic bag full of the aromatic herb.

The best and most economical way to get fresh herbs is to grow your own. Herbs can be expensive and variety limited at the grocery store. Luckily, most insects leave herbs alone, and once you get them planted they're very low maintenance. So just let them grow and cut from them as you wish.

There are various ways to preserve fresh herbs for later use. Susan washes and dries them, and puts them on baking sheets in the oven on the lowest temperature setting until they are very brittle, usually three or four hours. You can also tie them in bundles and let them dry naturally in a warm, dark, ventilated room. You may want to just put them whole in freezer bags after washing them. Make sure you dry them off before you place them in the bag.

Basil

While there are many different basil plants, sweet basil is the variety most often used for cooking. Its large green leaves are very aromatic and remind us of spaghetti sauce. When you notice your plant starting to bud or flower, pinch or cut the flowers off and chop them in your salad. They are a terrific addition of freshness. Basil is at its best before the flowers appear. It is best to cut from the plant early in the morning. In addition to wonderful flavor, basil also provides vitamin K, calcium, fiber, vitamin A, manganese, and magnesium. In Italy it was considered a symbol of love, but we love it as food! Use it in antipasto, or make some pesto! Basil pesto is delicious on crusty bread, in sauces, and especially in our Italian Bean Soup on page 175. Basil pairs well with many vegetables and seafood. Throughout history it has been used for its healing properties, including relief from nausea and flatulence, and it even repels insects. I have a few family members who need to eat more basil (and not for nausea), how about you? For a quick side salad, toss sliced grape or cherry tomatoes with chopped red onion, and then add some fresh mozzarella, freshly chopped basil, a little red wine vinegar, and some olive oil. Susan's husband loves this salad, and so will you!

Bay Leaf

Californian and Turkish are the two main types of bay leaves, which grow on a Mediterranean tree or shrub called bay laurel. Early Roman and Greek civilizations used the leaves in celebrations and thought they had magical properties. Most herbs are more potent when they're dried. Not so for bay leaves. Fresh ones are more flavorful and aromatic. Use bay leaves in soups, stews, and vegetable and rice dishes. They never soften, so always remove the leaves before serving your dish. Also, remember that using too many leaves can cause bitterness.

Black Pepper

Did you know black pepper comes from berries? The berries are dried and then ground for our common table pepper. Explorers were always looking for pepper to enhance the flavor of their less than fresh foods. Ancient people offered pepper to their gods, and it was even so valued it was used as money. A dash of pepper can aid digestion and reduce the effects of gas. As a bonus, you'll also get vitamin K, iron, and fiber!

Cayenne Pepper

A dash of this red pepper gives your dishes a zing! Start out with a little because you can always add more. It gives our immune systems a boost because of the beta-carotene and contains vitamins A, C, and B6, as well as manganese and fiber. Cayenne's high levels of capsaicin can reduce pain and inflammation, and even clear your nasal passages! If you like hot and spicy foods, has anyone ever told you that you're surely tearing up your stomach? Not true! Red pepper actually keeps ulcers from forming. And it can even boost your metabolism! Cayenne was used over 7,000 years ago. Explorers like Columbus hailed it as a very good substitute for black pepper.

Chives

These are the first of our herbs to appear in spring. Susan and I both grow onion chives, which produce lavender flowers. Garlic chives have white flowers. The flowers of either plant can be chopped into your salad. Rinse them very well, and soak them in salt water before using to make sure you get rid of the ants, which love these little flowers, too. Chives are a good source of iron. They are a fabulous infusion of color for potato, egg, or any creamy dish. They have a delicate flavor, and are a good source of vitamins A and C.

Cilantro

While chips and salsa may come to mind when you think of cilantro, another name for it is Chinese parsley! Early doctors used it for medicine because of its antibacterial properties, and it's known for its ability to freshen breath and to relieve flatulence and bloating. Are you surprised to learn that it can also kill salmonella? What a potent herb! Cilantro or coriander is one of the world's oldest spices, dating back to over 5000 BC. The ancient Romans and Greeks used it to enhance the flavor of their breads and to cure their meats. Cilantro provides us with fiber, iron, manganese, and magnesium, and has anti-inflammatory properties.

Cinnamon

Nothing is more comforting than the delicious scent of cinnamon. Did you know that brain function increases just by smelling cinnamon? Studies have shown that memory and attention increase with a whiff of cinnamon. It is the oldest spice known to man, and was used in medicines, beverages, flavorings, perfumes, and even to preserve bodies for burial. The bark on the cinnamon tree is rolled into sticks. You can use whole sticks or buy cinnamon in its most familiar form, ground. There's been a lot of attention lately to cinnamon's effect on lowering blood sugar. Studies show it helps with type 2 diabetes by helping the body react to insulin. The Chinese have long used it in tea to fight the common cold. Cinnamon gives us iron, fiber, and calcium.

Cumin

This smoky spice is native to Egypt, and the ancients used it for money and mummification. During the Middle Ages Europeans saw cumin as a symbol of love and devotion, and carried it with them to weddings. In addition, ancient Greeks and Romans used cumin in place of black pepper. You'll find cumin in Indian, Middle Eastern, and Mexican dishes. Try to buy it in seed form and then grind it using a mortar and pestle. Cumin is a good source of iron, giving us energy and helping to protect our immune systems. Cumin also contains manganese.

Dill

Native to the Mediterranean and parts of Russia and Africa, dill was used by ancient physicians who sometimes applied dill seed to wounds to promote healing. Dill was a sign of prosperity for the Greeks and Romans, who also thought it to have a calming effect on the stomach. Studies today have shown promise for dill's fighting power against certain carcinogens like smoke. Dill is easy to grow and provides us with calcium, fiber, and manganese. Known for its use in making pickles, it is also good with eggs, fish, potatoes, and in dips.

Ginger

A root vegetable, ginger gives us potassium, magnesium, copper, manganese, and vitamin B6. It has the ability to soothe the stomach and reduce gas. Did your mother ever give you ginger ale for an upset stomach? Your mother knew more than you thought. Ginger can reduce nausea and vomiting, and it also relieves inflammation. Studies of ginger show promise of its ability to kill ovarian cancer cells, and to help reduce the risk of tumors in the colon. Peel ginger and then slice, chop, or mince it. Add it near the end of cooking to retain its flavor and potency.

Oregano

Soldiers returning from Italy in the 20th century introduced the United States to oregano. Often called the pizza herb, it's a powerful antioxidant. The ancient Greeks and Romans made a laurel of oregano for brides and grooms, believing it to promote joy and happiness. Oregano is a close relative of marjoram, and is a good source of vitamins K, C, and A, as well as iron, fiber, manganese, calcium, and omega 3 fatty acids. In addition, studies have shown that oregano can slow the growth of certain bacteria, and may relieve respiratory symptoms during a cold. Adding it at the end of cooking time protects its potency.

Mint

Besides the obvious uses of giving us a fresh taste in toothpastes and gum, mint is full of nutrition, providing vitamins B2, C, and A, as well as iron, omega 3's, copper, fiber, potassium, and folate! Mint is also thought to have anti-cancer properties. Susan likes to chop it with parsley, basil, and chives for a nice blend of herbs to add to pasta salad. It can also be used to flavor meats and in teas. Mint has a calming effect on the stomach and can ease a spastic colon. Some studies have shown that the mere scent of mint can give you a lift and may make you more alert. So when you get that mid-afternoon slump at work, sniff some mint!

Mint can easily take over an herb garden, so you'll want to plant it where you have a lot of space or in a container by itself. Like most herbs, you can cut some off all summer and it will grow right back. Peppermint is stronger than spearmint, and spearmint is more often used in cooking. Early English colonists brought mint with them, and we have used it ever since as a flavoring for tea and other beverages.

Parsley

Unfortunately, a lot of parsley is thrown away or pushed to the edge of a plate due to its use as a garnish. Parsley as a garnish probably came about because it is thought to help with digestion and flatulence, and is a breath freshener. Undervalued, it's really a very good source of some key nutrients. Parsley is rich in vitamins K, C, and A, and is a good source of iron and folic acid. Parsley seed is hard and takes a while to germinate. An old legend says that parsley seed goes to the devil ten times before finally coming above ground. Once you get it started, your plant will return the next year. The next spring you'll need to replant. Wash parsley right before you use it, as it is very delicate. Add it at the end of your cooking time for optimal flavor and nutrition. Parsley was grown and consumed over 2,000 years ago in the Mediterranean region. Ancient Greeks made laurels of parsley for their athletes. Today curly and flat leaf parsleys are the most popular for cooking.

Rosemary

This is one of Susan's favorite herbs. While some may dislike the strong aroma, she loves it. Rosemary is really an evergreen, but it will not withstand frost. It even looks like something you picked off the yew bushes in front of your house. It is excellent with most meat and is wonderful baked into breads. Rosemary also pairs well with tomato and pasta dishes. Another tip Susan learned from her friend Sandy is to chop some rosemary into split pea soup. If you decide to try this, go easy with it at first to see how you like it. First cultivated in the Mediterranean region, ancient students would wear sprigs of it woven into their hair because they believed it would boost their memory. It was also customary to throw rosemary into graves during burial, and Shakespeare's Hamlet called out to Ophelia, "There's rosemary. That's for remembrance". Rosemary contains some fiber, calcium, and iron. It is thought to relieve headaches, calm the stomach, and help with circulation.

Sage

Sage has been consumed for thousands of years and, like many herbs, originated in the Mediterranean area. Ancient people used it to preserve their meat and for medicines, in cooking, and as a tea. Some believed it would provide immortality, as well as protection from witches. Recent studies show sage can boost memory, and that it has anti-cancer and anti-inflammatory properties. It's easy to grow and to preserve by drying. Try lightly sautéing sage leaves in olive oil, until they become delicately crunchy. Use fresh sage in stuffing, breads, and Italian cooking.

Salt

The next time you reach for a bag of chips, consider it not your fault! Studies are suggesting that we are born with a taste for salt, as are animals. Anybody ever buy a salt block for their horses, or for the deer in your yard? Sodium chloride (salt) is a mineral, which exists in many places throughout the world. Some salt deposits are beneath the ground and some are on the surface. There is even evidence of salt on the planet Mars! It's vital to our diet, and plays an important role in our lives. Did you ever wonder how sea salt, table salt and kosher salt differ? First, all salt is sea salt. Salt mines are simply ancient bodies of water that have dried up. Additives play a role in defining salt. Most salts have been treated with anti-caking additives and iodine. Iodine deficiency can cause thyroid problems, miscarriage, and can affect mental health. For this reason read the label when choosing to use kosher or sea salt, as some have been iodized and some have not. We read on *http://en.wikipedia.org* that Kosher salt gets its name not because it follows the guidelines for kosher foods as written in the Torah (nearly all salt is kosher, including ordinary table salt), but rather because of its use in making meats kosher, by helping to extract the blood from the meat. Because kosher salt grains are larger than regular table salt grains, when meats are coated in kosher salt the salt does not dissolve readily; the salt remains on the surface of the meat longer to draw fluids out of the meat. The biggest difference in salts is cost. As you might expect, table salt is the least expensive.

Thyme

Thyme is "chock full" of vitamin K and is also a great source of iron, manganese, calcium, and fiber. While it's been used for many years in cooking, ancient peoples thought of it as a symbol of bravery. They also used it to make a mouth rinse and in incense. It was grown in parts of Asia and the Mediterranean. It adds a slightly lemony zip to vegetables, meats, and sauces. Use thyme with vegetables, stews, tomato dishes, and meat. Thyme acts as an expectorant, and can be useful when fighting a cold.

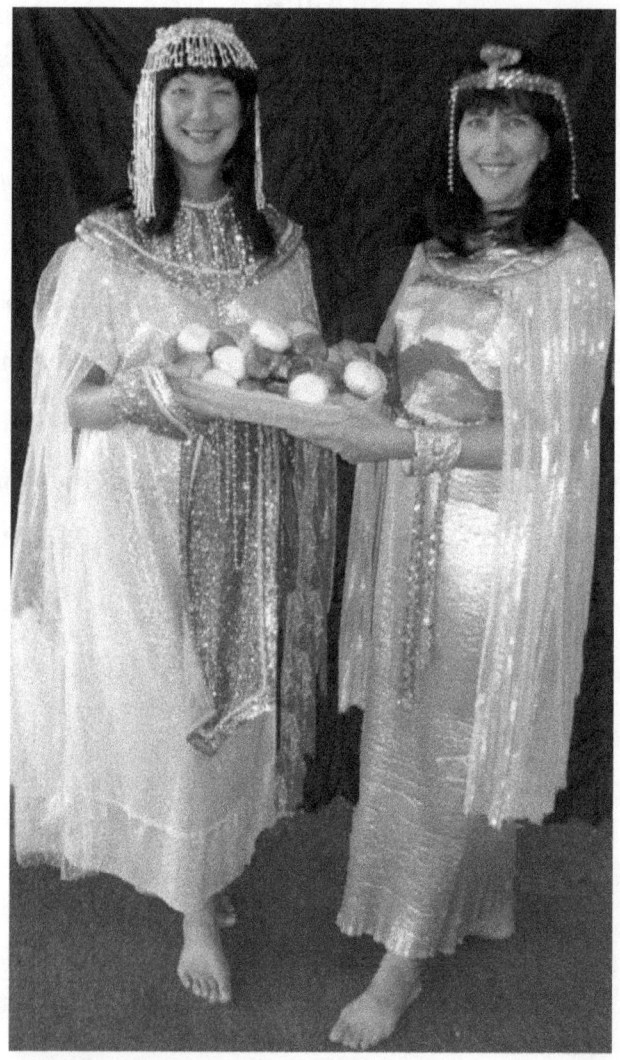

Photo 4 – Ancient Egyptians believed that eating mushrooms granted immortality. Maybe not, however, recent research shows many kinds of mushrooms clearly improve our health and protect us against disease.

The Magic Mushroom

Is there a fungus among us? You bet, and it's been around since prehistoric times. Mushrooms have no seeds and no roots, yet are a living organism, providing many nutrients. Ancient Egyptians believed that mushrooms granted immortality, according to the hieroglyphics left behind 4,600 years ago. The Pharaohs, who delighted in the flavor of mushrooms, decreed that they were food for royalty, and that no commoner could ever touch them. This, of course, enabled the Pharaohs to eat the entire supply of mushrooms. Several other cultures around the world believed that super human strength could be obtained by eating them, which would ultimately lead the soul to immortality. Some cultures even believed that eating mushrooms would help them find lost objects. The Romans called them "Food for the Gods."

For thousands of years, Eastern cultures have revered mushrooms as both food and medicine. It is said that there are more than 50 species with healing properties. Mushrooms, when used as medicine, are made into soup or tea, or taken as a tonic or elixir. Studies conducted over the past 30 years, mostly in Asia, have provided data suggesting that mushrooms or substances extracted from mushrooms may aid in the treatment of certain types of cancer, boost the immune system, and reduce the risk of coronary heart disease. Much of this research has focused on shiitake and maitake mushrooms. The first mushroom recipe we tried featured shiitake mushrooms. We found the recipe in Dr. Andrew Weil's book, <u>Eating Well for Optimum Health</u>, and modified it a bit. You will see our version of this recipe on page 121.

In China and Japan, the restorative powers of shiitake mushrooms are legendary. For centuries, they have been used to treat conditions such as colds and flu, poor circulation, upset stomachs, and even exhaustion. Scientific studies, conducted mainly in Japanese laboratories, have focused on two substances extracted from shiitake – lentinan and LEM. These substances are beta-glucans (mega-sugar molecules) that appear to kick immune system cells into action to help slow the spread of cancer cells and help fight infection.

In Japan, lentinan is used in combination with other types of chemotherapy in the treatment of lung cancer, melanoma, stomach cancer, breast cancer, and colorectal cancer. It is effective in helping suppress cancer recurrences, and in prolonging the lifespan of cancer patients. A shiitake extract called eritadenine is also being studied for its potential to reduce heart disease risk by reducing blood lipids and cholesterol levels.

Researchers in the United States are just beginning to take a serious look at the potential of mushrooms in disease control. At the Beckman Research Institute of the City of Hope in California, preliminary studies suggest that white mushrooms may play a role in treating or reducing the risk of breast cancer in post-menopausal women. A substance in white mushrooms was found to suppress breast cell proliferation by reducing the level of estrogen, a recognized factor in breast cancer development. The substance, yet to be identified, appears to inhibit the activity of aromatase, an enzyme involved in estrogen production.

Some early trials have also been published on mushrooms and prostate cancer risk reduction. A recent study at New York Medical College showed that maitake D-fraction destroyed prostate cancer cells in the test-tube. At the University of California at Davis, scientists are investigating the therapeutic effects of shiitake extracts on prostate cancer patients.

In the September 2008 issue of <u>Vegetarian Times</u>, Matthew Solan refers to research at the University of Illinois which found that raw and cooked maitake, shiitake, and white button mushrooms are rich in chitin, a dietary fiber known to lower cholesterol, and beta-glucan, which boosts the immune system.

This research is just the beginning of what promises to be an exciting journey into a fuller understanding of mushrooms and your health. Mushrooms may not grant us immortality as the ancient Egyptians believed, but recent research shows they clearly improve our health, protecting us from disease and reducing our risk of cardiovascular disease.

Cream of Mushroom Soup with Quinoa

- ½ cup quinoa
- 2 tablespoons extra virgin olive oil
- 1 small onion, chopped
- 1 clove garlic, minced
- 1 portabella cap, sliced or chopped
- 1 white button mushroom, sliced or chopped
- 1 14-ounce can low sodium chicken broth
- 1 cup 2% milk

Toast the quinoa in a skillet over medium heat about 5 minutes, stirring often. Add the olive oil, onion, garlic, and mushrooms. Cook for a few minutes, and then add chicken broth.

Let simmer for 15-20 minutes until quinoa is done. Transfer to a blender and blend until smooth.

Pour mixture back into skillet and add milk. Stir to combine. Garnish with fresh herbs.

<u>**Lunch Buddy Notes**</u> – Although this isn't a pretty soup, it makes up for its looks in good taste. It is rich, nutritious, full of flavor, and filling. You can easily double or even triple the recipe. In addition, it can be frozen and reheated.

Makes 4 servings.

Fettucine with Shiitake Mushrooms

- 1 pound whole wheat fettuccine or linguine
- ¼ cup extra virgin olive oil
- 2 cloves garlic, minced
- ½ pound shiitake mushrooms, sliced
- 2 tomatoes, chopped
- ¼ cup chopped basil
- 3 tablespoons finely chopped parsley

Cook pasta as directed on package and drain. Meanwhile, in fry pan over medium heat, cook garlic in hot olive oil until slightly browned; add mushrooms and tomatoes.

Cook for three to four minutes until vegetables are softened. Add basil and parsley.

Toss with hot pasta; serve with freshly grated Parmesan cheese.

<u>Lunch Buddy Notes</u> – If you plan to serve this for lunch the next day, don't toss with pasta. Store mushroom mixture, and pasta in separate containers. When you are ready to eat, first heat the pasta in the microwave or simply add hot water to the bag and drain. Then heat the mushroom mixture. Toss with hot pasta and serve with freshly grated Parmesan cheese.

<u>Food for Thought</u> – What does this lovely dish do for you? If you select Barilla Plus for your pasta, you get 17 grams of protein (30% of daily value), 7 grams of fiber (28% of daily value), and 360 mg of ALA Omega-3 (28% of daily value). Barilla Plus contains ground flaxseed, which is the highest

The Magic Mushroom

plant source of ALA omega-3, an essential fatty acid. The olive oil is, of course, a good source of monosaturated fat. Tomatoes are an excellent source of lycopene, and parsley is a good source of vitamins A and C, and calcium. And you already know the amazing benefits of the shiitake mushroom!

Did you know that the Greeks believed that parsley was a favorite herb of Hercules and wove it into victors' crowns at athletic festivals? They also wore it to absorb wine fumes and delay drunkenness, and they maintained that parsley seed worn in the hair would prevent baldness. Anyone know a balding husband we can try it out on?

Makes 4 to 6 servings.

Hot and Sour Soup

- 4 ounces fresh shiitake mushrooms, stems removed and caps thinly sliced
- 2 cloves garlic, minced
- 2 teaspoons extra virgin olive oil
- 28 ounces reduced-sodium chicken broth
- 2 tablespoons white vinegar or rice vinegar
- 2 tablespoons reduced-sodium soy sauce
- ½ teaspoon crushed red pepper flakes
- 1 cup chopped carrots
- 2 cups shredded cabbage
- 2 teaspoons water
- 1 tablespoon cornstarch
- 1 teaspoon sesame oil
- Sliced green onions

Cook mushrooms and garlic in hot oil (not smoking) 4 minutes. Stir occasionally. Add broth, vinegar, soy sauce, and red pepper. Stir and bring to boiling. Stir in cabbage and carrots. Bring to a boil, and then reduce heat. Let simmer for 5 minutes.

Stir cold water and cornstarch in a small bowl. Add to soup and simmer about 2 minutes, until thickened a little. Remove from heat and add sesame oil.

If you like them, sprinkle with green onions.

Makes 4 servings.

Mushroom Barley Soup

- 1 cup medium pearl barley
- 6 cups vegetable stock (we used organic vegetable stock; Dr. Weil makes his own vegetable stock)
- 1¼ cups onion, chopped
- 2 gloves garlic, minced
- 3 tablespoons extra virgin olive oil
- 1 pound fresh shiitake mushrooms, sliced (we used ¾ pound)
- 4 tablespoons dry sherry
- 4 tablespoons reduced-sodium soy sauce, or to taste
- 2 teaspoons dried dill weed or 2 tablespoons fresh dill

Rinse and drain the barley in a strainer. Cook the barley, covered, in 1½ cups of the broth in a large pot until tender. You may need to add broth as the barley absorbs it. Sauté the onions and garlic in the olive oil until they are nearly translucent.

Add the mushrooms and sherry and cook, uncovered, until the mushrooms are soft. Add the mushroom mixture to the barley with the remaining broth and the rest of the ingredients.

Reduce heat, cover, and bring the soup to a boil. Simmer for 20 minutes, and serve.

<u>**Lunch Buddy Notes**</u> – Make sure you do not heat any oil to the point of smoking and never breathe the smoke of heated or burning fat, which is highly toxic. This is another of Dr. Weil's recipes, which is as flavorful as it is healthful. This

wonderful soup can be served as an entrée for dinner parties. Your guests will love it! Just don't tell them it's a healthy dish, or they might not try it.

<u>*Food for Thought*</u> – If you think you don't like mushrooms, chase that thought right out of your head. The only mushrooms Susan had tried were fried mushrooms, and she didn't care for the gush of oil as she bit into them. Neither of us had eaten any mushrooms other than the common white mushroom and the wild morel so coveted by mushroom hunters everywhere. We have tried the recipes in this chapter using a variety of mushrooms, including shiitake, portabellas, cremini (baby bellas), and varied others and we LOVE them! So don't let your bias prevent you from trying a food which may magically improve your health. Listen to your elders, the Romans, and eat a food that is truly a "Food for the Gods."

According to Dr. Andrew Weil, this recipe provides 12 grams of fiber in an unrefined, whole grain, as well as monosaturated fat and micronutrients including immune-enhancing polysaccharides in the shiitake mushrooms. The recipe produces four servings, but for the serving size we like, it produced six servings with an extra bowl to enjoy after preparing it. I used my Food Saver, and put four servings in the freezer. It was just as delicious reheated in the microwave as fresh.

Makes 6 servings.

Mushrooms with Garlic

- 5 tablespoons extra virgin olive oil
- 1 pound white or cremini mushrooms, washed, trimmed, and cut into quarters
- Kosher salt
- 5 to 6 medium garlic cloves, minced (1½ tablespoons)
- 1 tablespoon sherry vinegar
- 2 tablespoons chopped fresh flat-leaf or curly parsley

Heat oil in a 12-inch skillet over medium high heat until hot. Add mushrooms, seasoning with ¾ teaspoon kosher salt. Stir to coat, then let cook undisturbed until the liquid released by the mushrooms evaporates and they are deep golden brown, approximately 5 to 7 minutes.

Continue sautéing, stirring occasionally, until most sides are nicely browned, 3 to 5 minutes longer.

Reduce heat to medium and add garlic. Cook just to soften, about 15 to 30 seconds. Add the vinegar and stir, scraping the bottom of the pan, until the vinegar evaporates, about 15 seconds. Remove the pan from the burner and toss in the parsley. Season with more salt to taste.

Makes 8 servings.

Mushroom and Spinach Frittata

- 4 cups spinach leaves
- 4 eggs or equivalent egg substitute
- ½ cup low fat cottage cheese
- ½ cup freshly grated Parmesan cheese
- 1 cup chopped mushrooms such as white, cremini, or portabella
- ½ cup chopped red onion
- ½ cup chopped red bell pepper
- ¼ teaspoon Italian seasoning
- Salt and pepper to taste

Preheat oven to 375° and spray a 9 inch pie plate with cooking spray. Stir all ingredients together and pour into pie plate.

Bake for 30 minutes or until browned on bottom and set. Let cool 10-15 minutes before serving.

<u>**Lunch Buddy Notes**</u> – What's a frittata? It's an Italian omelet, which is open faced and filled with hearty toppings, such as vegetables, meat, and cheese. We didn't include meat. You can easily prepare it ahead and reheat it when you're ready to eat it. We prepared our frittata with Egg Beaters, and couldn't tell the difference. It was delicious, satisfying, and made a beautiful presentation.

Makes 4 servings.

Mushroom and Vegetable Soup

- 2 tablespoons extra virgin olive oil
- 1 celery stalk, chopped
- 1 large carrot, chopped
- 2-3 cloves garlic, chopped
- 1 small onion, chopped
- 1 small zucchini unpeeled, halved, quartered, sliced
- 2 cups mushrooms of choice (portabellas, white button, shiitake)
- ¾ teaspoon thyme
- 4 cups low sodium vegetable broth
- 1 14.5-ounce can diced tomatoes
- 1 cup low sodium V-8
- Sea salt or kosher salt
- Black pepper

Sauté celery, carrot, garlic, onion, zucchini, and mushrooms in olive oil. Season with kosher salt or sea salt, thyme, and black pepper. Add vegetable broth, tomatoes, and V-8.

Cook over medium heat and bring to a boil, then reduce heat and simmer for about 30 minutes or until vegetables are tender.

Makes 5 servings.

Pasta with Cremini

- 3 tablespoons extra virgin olive oil
- ⅓ cup chopped onion
- ½ teaspoon ground coriander
- ½ teaspoon chili powder
- 1 teaspoon minced garlic
- ¼ teaspoon black pepper
- 1 teaspoon sea salt
- 1 teaspoon lemon juice
- ¼ cup Marsala Cooking Wine
- 1 teaspoon sugar
- 1 tablespoon soy sauce
- ½ pound fresh cremini, sliced
- 5 ounces Healthy Harvest Whole Wheat Blend Pasta Extra Wide Noodles
- 1½ tablespoons cornstarch, mixed with ⅓ cup cold water

Heat olive oil slowly in a large skillet and add onion. Over medium high heat, sauté the onion until just translucent, one to two minutes.

Add ½ cup water to the skillet. Add seasonings, lemon juice, wine, sugar, and soy sauce, and stir. Turn heat to low and add the mushrooms. Simmer covered for 30 minutes. Meanwhile, add the noodles to a large pot of boiling, lightly salted water (about 4 quarts). Cook until just slightly firm. Drain.

While the noodles are cooking, add the cornstarch mixture to the mushrooms, stir, and heat just until thickened. If eating right away, place the noodles on a serving dish and spoon the mushrooms and sauce over.

<u>Lunch Buddy Notes</u> – This dish can be easily reheated. We froze the mushroom mixture and noodles in separate bags. When you freeze the noodles, we recommend just using the sealing feature on your Food Saver. If you use the vacuum and seal, the noodles stick together in a big clump. The bag lays flatter if you simply seal it. We divided the noodles, and placed them on two serving dishes. We spooned the mushroom sauce over each, and reheated. The original recipe called for butter and salt. We lightened the recipe by using extra virgin olive oil and sea salt. The dish is so rich and delicious; you will think there is a whole stick of butter in it.

In addition to boosting immunity and suppressing some forms of cancer, mushrooms are high in fiber, low in calories, and free of sodium, fat, and cholesterol. The exotic shiitake is high in fiber and protein, with lots of flavor. The white cultivated mushroom has lots of potassium, which helps lower blood pressure. Fiber helps lower the risk of developing certain conditions such as heart disease, cancer, and diabetes.

In addition, mushrooms contain large amounts of an antioxidant called L-ergothioneine. It's believed that fungi are the only foods containing this compound.

The Healthy Harvest Noodles provide 6 grams (24%) of dietary fiber, 7 grams of protein, 30% of thiamin, 20% of niacin, 15% riboflavin, 10% of iron, and 30% of folate. These noodles add a nutritional punch to this dish.

The Magic Mushroom

So don't give up your noodles ... just replace them with healthy ones! They are only a shade darker than the noodles made with white flour, and you may think they taste better. Just close your eyes, and take a bite!

Makes 4 servings.

Porcini Risotto

- 2 ounces dried porcini mushrooms
- 14.5 ounces organic beef broth
- 4 tablespoons extra virgin olive oil
- 1 onion, diced
- 1 garlic clove, minced
- 2 cups Arborio rice
- ½ cup dry white wine
- ¾ cup freshly grated Parmesan

Place mushrooms in medium bowl, cover with hot water and soak for 30 minutes. Remove mushrooms from the water and chop into large pieces, reserving liquid. Strain liquid.

Combine liquid, beef broth, and water to equal 6 cups. In a small saucepan, bring to a low boil.

In a stock pot, heat olive oil. Sauté onion and garlic until translucent. Add rice, stir, and cook about 2 minutes. Add wine, and cook until liquid is nearly gone. Stir in mushrooms and 1 cup warm broth mixture.

Continue adding warm broth ½ cup at a time, stirring constantly. Cook at a simmer until al dente, about 20 minutes. Use only as much liquid as is needed. You may wish to save the rest for other recipes. Remove from heat and stir in remaining olive oil and Parmesan. Let sit 10 minutes.

The Magic Mushroom

Lunch Buddy Notes – What's risotto? If you grew up with Minute Rice, like Susan and I, you might not know. Risotto is a traditional Italian dish made with Arborio or other suitable rice. It's one of the most common ways of cooking rice in Italy. Risotto originated in North Italy, where rice paddies are abundant. It's a very creamy rice dish, which is cooked by adding liquid periodically throughout the cooking time.

Makes 6 servings.

Wild Rice and Mushroom Soup

- 1 small onion, finely chopped
- 2 teaspoons extra virgin olive oil
- 2 garlic cloves, minced
- 12 ounces fresh wild mushrooms (morel, porcini, shiitake, or portabella), cleaned and sliced
- 1 carrot, finely chopped
- 1 rib celery, finely chopped
- 6 cups (48 ounces) organic low sodium chicken or vegetable broth
- ⅓ cup wild rice
- 1 teaspoon thyme
- ¼ cup red wine (optional)

Sauté onion in oil until translucent in a large pot. Add garlic, mushrooms, carrot, and celery. Cook covered until vegetables are soft, about three minutes.

Add broth, rice, thyme, and wine, if desired. Bring to a boil, reduce heat, cover, and simmer about an hour until rice is tender.

Lunch Buddy Notes – Here you are at the end of the mushroom chapter. How many of you are now mycophagists? You probably didn't know there is a noun to describe people who love mushrooms. That's because if you love mushrooms, you are a special person. Mushrooms have been revered for thousands of years, and it appears our ancestors were pretty wise about their magical properties.

Makes 6 servings.

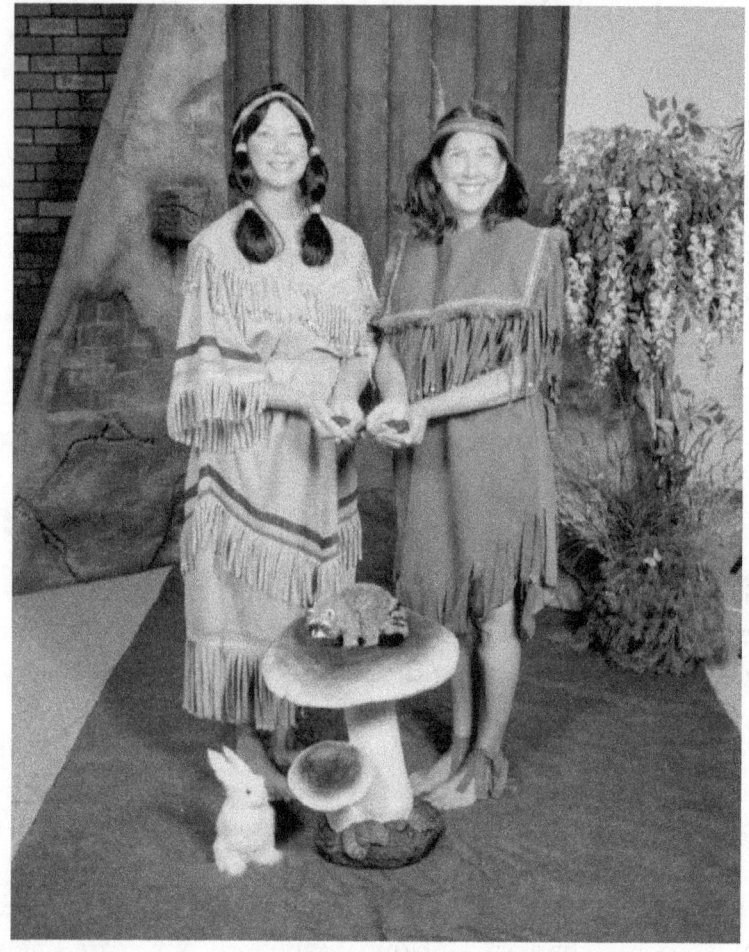

Photo 5 – Native Americans were the first to enjoy wild rice, more than 12,000 years ago.

Go Go Grains

Not all grains are created equal. Surprisingly, even white sandwich bread contains fiber. However, you would have to eat 11 pieces to satisfy your daily recommended value. Add some milk or water to those 11 pieces of white bread in your stomach, and imagine how you might feel.

I know a young woman who ate a whole tube of raw refrigerated biscuits, and in the middle of the night her stomach pains sent her to the local emergency department. I imagine those 11 pieces of soppy white bread in your stomach might do the same to you. So let's be sensible, learn about whole grains, and begin incorporating them in our diet.

Why do we need to eat foods rich in fiber, such as whole grains? As part of a healthy diet, they are believed to:

*Reduce the risk of coronary heart disease.

*Reduce constipation.

*Help with weight management.

*Help reduce blood cholesterol levels.

*Boost your immune system.

Go Go Grains

Researchers at the University of Minnesota conducted a study which demonstrated that eating just three daily servings of whole grains can reduce your risk of heart disease by 25 to 36 percent, stroke by 37 percent, and type 2 diabetes by 21 to 27 percent.

What's the difference between a whole grain and a refined grain? The USDA website, *www.mypyramid.gov* explains that whole grains contain the entire grain kernel – the bran, germ, and endosperm. Brown rice, whole wheat flour, oats, barley, bulgur, and buckwheat groats are examples of whole grains. Refined grains have been milled, a process which removes the bran and germ. The purpose of milling is to give the grains a finer texture and improve their shelf life. Unfortunately, milling also removes dietary fiber, iron, and many B vitamins. Refined grains include white flour, white bread, and white rice. Most refined grains are enriched, meaning that some B vitamins and iron are added back after processing. The fiber, however, cannot be added back to enriched grains.

What have we done to our wholesome sources of fiber? We have stripped them of their best qualities, in order to provide a convenient, economical food source.

Generations of Americans have grown up eating only white bread and rice. They seem to believe brown is a bad color. If your family is like mine, just bring out a bowl of brown rice, and watch the facial expressions. Most are unwilling to try these foreign-looking grains. With food, unfamiliarity seems to breed contempt.

Quinoa

Now, clear your mind of all its prejudices and let's take a journey back in time beginning 5,000 years ago in the vast Inca Empire. We are going to introduce you to a tiny grain the Incas called quinoa (keen-wa), meaning "The Mother Grain." Quinoa was so sacred that each year the mighty Inca ruler himself planted the first row with a solid gold spade. This tiny grain is no bigger than a mustard seed, yet it once fed an ancient civilization which stretched from the seacoast of Chile to the snow-capped peaks of the Peruvian Andes.

Quinoa, as rugged as the Andes, has flourished in cultivation for thousands of years. The Quinoa Corporation now designates it as "The Supergrain of the Future." If you can't find it in your supermarket, just head to the nearest health food store. For your extra ten minutes, you will be purchasing an excellent source of iron and phosphorus, and a good source of fiber and riboflavin. A nutritional bonus is that quinoa contains more protein than any other grain, according to the Quinoa Corporation website, *www.quinoa.net*.

Barley

Get your suitcase packed for another trip ... this time we're going back to 8000 BC, when barley was first used, according to studies by agronomists. Barley, one of the most ancient of cultivated plants, is even mentioned several times in the Bible. The Hebrews cultivated and consumed barley. It was also grown by the ancient Egyptians, Greeks, Romans, and Chinese. Roman gladiators dined on barley for a source of energy and strength. While the Pharaohs were munching on mushrooms, enslaved Egyptians ate barley bread as their sole sustenance. Think that you can do without carbohydrates, including whole grains? Take a look at the pyramids. Just think what you might be able to accomplish if you include whole grains and barley in your diet.

Unfortunately for our health, most of the barley now grown is used to make beer and whiskey, or for animal feed.

Take our advice. Eating barley is much better for you than drinking it. Just one quarter of a cup of pearled barley provides eight grams of dietary fiber. Barley is also a good source of iron, selenium, and niacin.

Brown Rice

Here we go again ... and don't forget your chopsticks. This time we're heading to southern China. Radiocarbon dating of strata containing grains of rice tells us it was cultivated as far back as 7,000 years ago.

Today in China the word for rice is the same as the word for food. In Thailand when you call your family to a meal you say, "Eat rice"; and in Japan the word for cooked rice is the same as the word for meal. The shower of rice most newlyweds experience comes from an ancient ritual symbolizing fertility and the blessing of many children. Today it symbolizes prosperity and abundance.

The Japanese believe that soaking rice before cooking releases the life energy and gives the eater a more peaceful soul. There is a mystical aura in Japan surrounding the planting, harvesting, and preparation of rice.

Parents tell young Chinese girls who leave rice in their bowls that each grain of rice they leave represents a pock mark on the face of their future husbands. In China instead of greeting each other with "How are you?" they say "Have you had your rice today?" The expected response is "Yes."

There are perhaps as many as 40,000 varieties of rice grown on every continent, except Antarctica. Surprisingly, the United States is the twelfth largest rice producer worldwide, and the second largest exporter of rice. The average person in Burma eats 500 pounds of rice a year, which equates to 1¼ pounds per day, while the average American eats only twenty-five pounds of rice per year, with four pounds of that figure attributed to the rice used to brew beer. Although Americans eat twice as much rice as we did ten years ago, we still export about half of the rice we grow.

Rice is high in complex carbohydrates, contains almost no fat, is cholesterol free, and is low in salt. Brown rice has five times more vitamin E, three times more magnesium, and twice as much fiber as white rice. Rice contains all eight essential amino acids, and when combined with beans, provides a complete protein. Rice is a good choice for people with wheat allergies or digestive problems because it is gluten free and easily digestible.

Wild Rice

Grab your rubber boots, and get ready to travel back again, this time to 12,000 years ago. You'll need the boots to get around in the lake and river bed areas where this cereal grain grows. You may be wondering why wild rice isn't included in the rice section. Actually wild rice is not rice at all, but is the seed of aquatic grasses growing in shallow water.

When early Europeans first settled around the Great Lakes area of North America, the inhabitants already living there considered the "wild" varieties of lake and river wild rice to be "A Gift from the Great Spirit ... the Creator Himself". Native Americans rowed their canoes into a stand of plants, and used wooden sticks called knockers to bend the ripe grain heads and thresh the seeds into the canoe. The size of the knockers was actually proscribed by tribal and state laws. Early French explorers called it Riz Sauvage (wild rice) or Folles Avoines (wild oats).

Today it is often called "The Caviar of all Grains." Its sweet tasting nutty texture is cherished by many, and is included in many a gourmet meal. Wild rice is high in protein, the amino acid lysine, and dietary fiber. On top of all that, it is also low in fat. Like true rice, it does not contain gluten. It is a good source of potassium, phosphorus, thiamine, riboflavin, and niacin. Wild rice is often combined with true rice due to its comparatively high cost and chewy texture.

By the way, wild rice isn't just important as a food source for us ... it also provides a unique habitat for fish and waterfowl. So grab a fish and some wild rice, and let's get ready for our next journey.

Oats

Oats persisted as a weed-like plant in fields of other cultivated crops for centuries prior to domestication. While the Romans scored an A on mushrooms, they flunked the oat test. The Greeks and Romans both considered oats to be nothing more than a diseased version of wheat. The Romans fed the oats to their horses, and scorned the "oat-eating barbarians". These barbarians were the pesky Germanic tribes who eventually toppled the West Roman Empire. The Romans also tried several times to defeat the

Scots (who were big oat eaters), and failed each time they tried.

Our present cultivated oats may have developed as a mutation from wild oats in Asia Minor or southeastern Europe not long before the birth of Christ. Oats were first brought to North America in 1602. In 1786 George Washington sowed 580 acres in oats. By the mid 1800's cultivation had moved west to the middle and upper Mississippi Valley, where most of the oats in the United States are grown today.

Why should we eat oats? Oats contain more soluble fiber than any other grain. Soluble fiber moves slowly through your body, and makes you feel full longer, while also slowing the absorption of glucose. Clever oat eaters, who skip the sugary processed cereals, sweet rolls, and donuts, will also avoid those nasty sugar highs and lows. You probably have read that oats lower cholesterol. Wonder how that works? The soluble fiber in oats inhibits the re-absorption of bile into the system, forcing your liver to get its cholesterol fix from your blood, which lowers your blood-serum cholesterol. Susan and I both eat steel cut oats for breakfast nearly every day. We'll talk about these in a bit.

After hearing about all the great things oats can do for us, are you surprised that less than 5% of the oats now grown commercially are for human consumption? Centuries after the Romans fed oats to their horses, even today the chief value of oats remains as a crop grown for livestock, especially horses. My daughter, Kate, lives on a 35 head horse farm in Springfield, Illinois. Occasionally, I help her feed the horses their oats (grown at the farm), along with processed feeds made by ADM Alliance. You should hear the horses munching on their grains. Horses weigh hundreds of pounds more than you, and yet grains are their primary food (or fuel). So take a lesson from Mr. Ed, and eat your grains. You just might find yourself galloping off to work in the morning!

Before we heard of steel cut oats, Susan and I ate a lot of instant oatmeal. Sorry to report that, although convenient, instant oatmeal contains a lot of sugar and not as much fiber as steel cut oats or even our old standby, Quaker Oats. Steel cut oats are no more trouble to prepare. Just boil some water, add your oats and cook for about 15 minutes. Make them ahead and you will have all your breakfasts for the week. When you reheat in the microwave, simply add a little water or milk for moisture. You can add fruit, such as blueberries, strawberries, or bananas, or honey, peanut butter, brown sugar, or even a little maple syrup. After a few months of eating steel cut oats or Quaker rolled oats for breakfast, don't be surprised when you see a significant drop in your cholesterol.

Whole Wheat

Like wild rice, wheat was originally a wild grass. There is evidence that wheat first grew in Mesopotamia, as well as in the river valleys in the Middle East, close to 10,000 years ago. Now that's a lot of generations! Ever hear of Mesopotamia? When we were young, Dad nicknamed my sister "Mesopotamia" (for obvious reasons). I never realized until much later that Mesopotamia actually means "the land between the two rivers", and was located in the present Middle-Eastern country of Iraq. It is often called the "cradle of civilization" because it was here the first civilization formed in the year 3500 BC. This advanced civilization learned to control the flooding rivers and grew barley, wheat, flax, and sesame, as well as a multitude of fruits and vegetables.

Egyptians were the first to discover how to make yeast-leavened breads between 2000 and 3000 BC. Wheat is the only grain with enough gluten content to make a raised loaf of bread, and quickly became the favored grain of those times. The workers who built the pyramids in Egypt were actually paid in bread.

Although today wheat is grown on more acres in the United States than any other grain, it is not native to the United States. It was brought to the United States by Russian Mennonites, who settled in Kansas in the late 1800's, and brought with them Turkey Red winter wheat. Today wheat is grown in 42 states, and is used in more foods than is any other cereal grain.

Popcorn

Grab a bowl and a movie … we're taking another trip, one which will take us back to 2500 BC to a bat cave in Mexico, where the oldest ears of popcorn were found in 1948. Cachise Indians are thought to have grown and eaten popcorn. A funeral urn from 300 AD, also found in Mexico, shows a picture of a maize god with a primitive popcorn headdress. Popcorn kernels more than 1,000 years old have been found in tombs on the east coast of Peru, some of which still pop.

Most of us have heard the story that the English colonists were introduced to popcorn at the first Thanksgiving feast in Plymouth, Massachusetts. It is told that one of the chief's brothers arrived with a goodwill gift of popped corn in a deerskin bag. The colonists then came up with the idea of eating popcorn with milk and sugar, thus creating the first breakfast cereal.

Columbus found the natives in the West Indies eating popcorn, as well as using it for decoration. Cortez discovered, after invading Mexico in 1519, that popcorn was just as important to the Aztecs, who used it for decorating their ceremonial headdresses and necklaces, as well as for food.

Are you surprised to find out that popcorn is a whole grain? Three cups count as one equivalent ounce of whole grain. So go light on the butter and salt, and feed yourself a wholesome whole grain food. And don't let the bats scare you off.

Barley and Lentil Stew with Mushrooms

- 2 tablespoons extra virgin olive oil
- 1 tablespoon chopped garlic
- 1 small onion, chopped
- 1 tablespoon chopped fresh sage or ½ teaspoon dried
- 1 stalk celery, chopped
- 1 carrot, sliced
- 2 cups assorted sliced or chopped white mushrooms
- 2 32-ounce containers low sodium vegetable broth
- 2 bay leaves
- ½ cup fresh whole basil leaves or 1 teaspoon dried basil
- 1 teaspoon dried savory
- ¾ cups of pearl barley
- ¾ cup lentils
- Salt and pepper to taste

In a soup pan, sauté the garlic, onion, sage, celery, and carrot in the olive oil for about 10 minutes. Add mushrooms and sauté another 5 minutes. Add broth, bay leaves, basil, savory, and barley. Bring to a boil, then reduce heat to low, and simmer 20-25 minutes. Add lentils and simmer another 20 minutes until lentils are done. If you prefer a soup rather than a stew, use three 32-ounce containers of the broth.

Lunch Buddy Notes – This stew is loaded with fiber, folate, and iron.

Makes 8 to 10 servings.

Barley Stuffed Bell Peppers

- 4 bell peppers (any color or combination of colors)
- Extra virgin olive oil
- ½ onion, chopped
- 1 large clove of garlic, minced
- 1 large or 2 small carrots, sliced
- ½ cup pearled barley
- 1 15.5-ounce can diced or stewed tomatoes or 10-12 fresh Italian tomatoes peeled, seeded, and diced
- 2 cups vegetable or chicken broth
- Assorted fresh herbs chopped, such as basil, parsley, chives, mint, or sage

Wash and split peppers and remove seeds. Steam them either in a steamer or in a casserole dish in the microwave, leaving them still firm but softened.

Sauté the onion, garlic, and carrots in the olive oil in a large skillet for 10 minutes or so. Add the barley and toast it for five minutes. Add the tomatoes and broth and bring to a boil. Cover, reduce heat, and simmer until barley is done. Stir in chopped herbs. Stuff peppers with barley and reheat just before eating.

<u>**Lunch Buddy Notes**</u> – You can serve immediately, or the peppers keep very well for a few days in the refrigerator. They can be reheated in a microwave.

Makes 4 servings.

Confetti Rice

- 1 tablespoon butter
- 2 tablespoons extra virgin olive oil
- 1 carrot, finely chopped
- 2 celery ribs, finely chopped (pick ribs with lots of celery leaves)
- 1 small onion, finely chopped
- 1 large garlic clove, minced
- ¼ cup green pepper, finely chopped
- ¼ cup red pepper, finely chopped
- 1 cup sliced mushrooms, any variety
- 2 pinches of kosher salt
- Sprinkle of black pepper
- ¾ cup brown rice
- ½ teaspoon herbs de Provence
- 1 can vegetable broth (14 ounces), organic preferred
- 1 can chicken stock (14 ounces), organic preferred

Over medium heat, sauté vegetables, seasonings, herbs, and rice in butter and oil for about 10 minutes. Add the broths and bring to a boil. Reduce heat to simmer and cover. Simmer, stirring occasionally, for 1 hour and 10 minutes.

<u>**Lunch Buddy Notes**</u> – Herbs de Provence is a general mixture of dried herbs that grow naturally in the Provence area of France. The blend includes basil, marjoram, summer savory, thyme, bay leaf, fennel, and occasionally lavender. If you prefer to skip the butter, just increase the olive oil to three tablespoons.

Makes 4 servings.

Hearty Barley Soup

- ½ cup chopped onions
- ½ cup chopped leeks
- ½ cup chopped celery
- ½ cup chopped carrots
- ¼ cup olive oil
- 6 ½ cups organic chicken broth
- ⅔ cup pearl barley
- ¾ teaspoon dried thyme
- ¾ teaspoon dried marjoram
- 4 sprigs fresh parsley or several sprinkles of freeze dried parsley
- 1 large potato, peeled and diced
- 1 cup skim milk

Chop vegetables into medium large chunks, or small if you prefer. Sauté onion, leeks, celery, and carrots in olive oil for 10 minutes in a large soup pot. Add chicken broth, pearl barley, thyme, marjoram, and parsley. Then bring to a boil, reduce heat, and simmer, partially covered, for one hour. Add broth as needed.

Add the diced potato and simmer about 40 minutes longer, or until potatoes and barley are tender, yet not mushy. Add the milk, and freshly ground pepper to taste.

Garnish with fresh parsley.

Lunch Buddy Notes – You can substitute fresh herbs, if available. Instead of ¾ teaspoon, use ¾ tablespoon.

Makes 6 servings.

Mushroom Barley Bake

- ¼ cup extra virgin olive oil
- 1 medium onion, diced
- 2 garlic cloves, minced
- 1 cup uncooked pearl barley
- ½ cup pine nuts
- 2 green onions, thinly sliced
- 1 cup sliced fresh cremini mushrooms
- ½ cup chopped fresh or freeze dried parsley
- ¼ teaspoon sea salt
- ⅛ teaspoon pepper
- 30 ounces vegetable broth (organic preferably)

Preheat oven to 350°. Sauté onion, garlic, barley, and pine nuts in olive oil until barley is lightly browned.

Add green onions, mushrooms, and parsley and stir. Season with salt and pepper; then place in a 2 quart casserole dish. Stir in the vegetable broth.

Bake one hour and 15 minutes in a preheated oven, until liquid has been absorbed and barley is tender.

<u>**Lunch Buddy Notes**</u> – You may use cremini (baby bellas) or regular white mushrooms in this recipe. You'll be adding 7 grams of fiber and 7.5 grams of protein to your diet with just one serving of this delicious dish. The original recipe called for 1/4 cup of butter and regular salt, which we changed to the healthier extra virgin olive oil and sea salt.

Makes 4 servings.

Mushroom Rice Bake

- 2 cups uncooked brown rice
- ½ cup extra virgin olive oil
- 1 cup finely chopped celery
- 1 cup finely chopped Vidalia (or other sweet) onion
- 2 cups sliced fresh cremini or white mushrooms
- 4 cups organic chicken broth
- ⅔ cup water
- 3 tablespoons soy sauce
- 4 tablespoons fresh or 2 tablespoons dried parsley leaves

Sauté rice in olive oil for 2 to 3 minutes. Add celery and onion, and cook for 2 more minutes, stirring occasionally. Add mushrooms, and heat until celery is tender.

Spray a three quart casserole dish with olive oil; then place mixture in the dish. Add the broth, water, soy sauce, and parsley, then stir.

Cover. Bake at 350° for approximately one hour, until liquid is absorbed and rice is tender.

<u>Lunch Buddy Notes</u> – Reheats well in the microwave. Be sure to check the rice for doneness, as brown rice takes longer to cook than white rice.

Makes 12 servings.

Quinoa Pilaf

- 3 tablespoons pine nuts
- 2 large onions, chopped
- 6 cloves garlic, minced
- 2 tablespoons extra virgin olive oil
- 1 red or green bell pepper, chopped
- 4 teaspoons cumin
- 2 cups quinoa
- 1 cup fresh basil leaves, chopped
- 1 can corn (14.5 ounces)
- 3 ½ cups water

Preheat oven to 350°. Spread pine nuts on a baking sheet. Toast for 3 minutes. Take out and set aside. In a large saucepan, sauté onions and garlic in the olive oil for a few minutes. Add the pepper and cumin and continue to sauté.

Add quinoa, basil, corn, and water to saucepan. Bring to a boil, then turn heat to low, and cover. Cook until quinoa is done, about 20 minutes. Add salt and pepper to taste. Sprinkle with toasted pine nuts when serving.

Lunch Buddy Notes – If fresh basil is not available, use ⅓ cup dried basil.

Makes 4 to 6 servings.

Roasty Toasty Barley Stew

- 2 bell peppers, any color
- 3 yellow and green zucchinis
- 2 medium onions
- 4 carrots
- Herbs (may use oregano, herbs de Provence or Fines herbs)
- Extra virgin olive oil
- 1 head of garlic, peeled, chopped, and reserved
- 1 cup pearl barley
- 1 ½ 32-ounce cartons of vegetable broth, chicken broth or a combination of the two
- 1 can of diced tomatoes, 14.5 or 15 ounces

Preheat oven to 425°. Cut vegetables into bite-size chunks and place on a cookie sheet. Sprinkle them with your favorite dried herbs, such as herbs de Provence, or Fines herbs. Drizzle the vegetables with extra virgin olive oil and roast for about 30 minutes, or until tender and caramelized. Sprinkle with garlic when almost done. Remove from oven.

While the vegetables are roasting, put enough extra virgin olive oil in a very large saucepan to lightly coat the bottom. Add 1 cup of pearl barley and stir occasionally over medium heat. Continue to toast the barley for about ten minutes. Add one and a half 32-ounce containers of vegetable broth or chicken broth, or a combination of the two. Stand back because the barley will splatter when you add the liquid. Add the diced tomatoes and the roasted veggies.

Bring the stew to a boil, and then reduce heat to a simmer until barley is done.

Makes 6 servings.

Lunch Buddy Notes – Mushrooms are a delicious addition to the roasted vegetables. Use any combination of your favorite vegetables, broths, and herbs.

Summer Garden Quinoa

- Extra virgin olive oil
- 1 or 2 cloves garlic
- 1 small onion
- 1 bell pepper
- 8 small or 4 large fresh tomatoes
- ½ cup quinoa
- Sea salt and black pepper
- ¼ cup chopped fresh herbs (whatever you have in your garden, such as mint, chives, basil, or parsley)

Chop garlic, onion, pepper, and tomatoes. Sauté in olive oil in skillet for 10-15 minutes. Add quinoa and cook 15 minutes more. Then add herbs and stir.

<u>**Lunch Buddy Notes**</u> – This is a wonderful summer dish, and a great way to utilize your fresh herbs. If you don't have a garden, plant some herbs in your flowerbeds. You'll be surprised how pretty they look, and how much you'll enjoy cooking with them.

Makes 4 servings.

Tomato Oatmeal Soup

- 2 onions, chopped
- 6 cloves crushed garlic
- 8 tablespoons olive oil
- 2 cans low-sodium stewed tomatoes (14.5 ounces each)
- 1 tablespoon fresh or freeze dried oregano
- 1 tablespoon fresh or freeze dried basil
- 8 cups water
- ¼ teaspoon pepper, or to taste
- 1 ½ cups rolled oats

Sauté onion and garlic in olive oil, until onion is tender. Add tomatoes (not drained), water, oregano, basil, and pepper. Simmer.

Meanwhile, toast rolled oats in a heavy sauce pan, stirring till they are slightly brown. Stir oats into soup and cook for 6 to 10 minutes.

Lunch Buddy Notes – Don't like oatmeal? Here's a delicious way to eat your oats. Like us, you may have never thought of putting oats in soup. We found the original recipe on *www.allrecipescom*, and changed it just a bit, substituting olive oil for margarine, adding oregano and basil, and leaving out the salt. Once you begin cooking with herbs, you will find there is plenty of flavor without adding salt. Your blood pressure will thank you later. And your cholesterol will thank you for eating oats.

Makes 8 servings.

Vegetarian Chili with Brown Rice

- 1 15 ½-ounce can red kidney beans, rinsed and drained
- 1 15-ounce can great northern beans, rinsed and drained
- 1 14 ½-ounce can low-sodium tomatoes, undrained and cut up
- 1 8-ounce can tomato sauce
- 1 cup water
- ¾ cup chopped green pepper
- ½ cup chopped onion
- 1 tablespoon chili powder
- 1 teaspoon sugar
- 1 tablespoon snipped fresh basil or 1/2 teaspoon dried basil, crushed
- ½ teaspoon ground cumin
- ¼ teaspoon sea salt
- Dash ground red pepper
- 2 cloves garlic, minced
- 2 cups hot cooked brown rice

Combine kidney beans, great northern beans, undrained tomatoes, tomato sauce, water, green pepper, onion, chili powder, sugar, basil, cumin, sea salt, ground red pepper, and garlic in a large saucepan. Bring to a boil and reduce heat. Cover and simmer for 15 minutes. Stir occasionally.

Top each serving of chili with ½ cup hot cooked brown rice.

Makes 6 to 8 servings.

Go Go Grains

Lunch Buddy Notes – We usually double this recipe and freeze 6 servings for easy lunches during busy times. We use food saver bags, freezing the chili and rice separately. After topping the chili with the rice, you can sprinkle on a little cheese, if you like.

Wild Rice and Mushrooms

- 1 cup dried porcini or shiitake mushrooms
- 2 ½ cups water
- 1 cup wild rice
- ½ cup freshly squeezed orange juice
- ¼ cup dry sherry
- ½ cup slice carrots
- 2 tablespoons chopped fresh parsley or 2 teaspoons dried parsley
- Sea salt or natural soy sauce to taste
- ½ cup finely chopped walnuts or pecans

Soak the dried mushrooms in water to cover until they are soft. Squeeze them out, reserving liquid and slice.

Wash the wild rice in cold water and place in a pot with the mushroom-soaking liquid (minus sediment) and enough additional cold water to total two cups. Add the orange juice, sherry, and carrots. Bring to a boil. Reduce heat, cover and simmer for 30 minutes.

Add the mushrooms and continue cooking until rice is tender and all the liquid is absorbed. Add the chopped or dried parsley, and salt or soy sauce to taste. Stir in the finely chopped nuts.

<u>**Lunch Buddy Notes**</u> – This is a Dr. Andrew Weil recipe. We signed up to receive his recipe of the day, and this is one we especially like.

Makes 4 servings.

Wild Rice, Pine Nuts, and Cranberries

- 2 bunches scallions (green onions), rinsed, stems removed
- 2 tablespoons extra virgin olive oil, divided
- 1 5-ounce package wild rice
- 2 ounces sweetened, dried cranberries or cran-raisins
- 1 ¾ ounces pine nuts, toasted
- ⅓ cup finely chopped parsley
- Sea salt and pepper to taste

Slice scallions diagonally into ¼ inch pieces. Heat one tablespoon olive oil on moderately high heat. Add scallions and sauté one to two minutes, stirring frequently. Set aside.

Prepare wild rice according to package cooking instructions. When finished, remove lid from pan, gently stir in the scallions, sweetened dried cranberries, toasted pine nuts, finely chopped parsley, and one tablespoon of remaining oil. Heat for one minute. Serve warm.

Makes 4 to 6 servings.

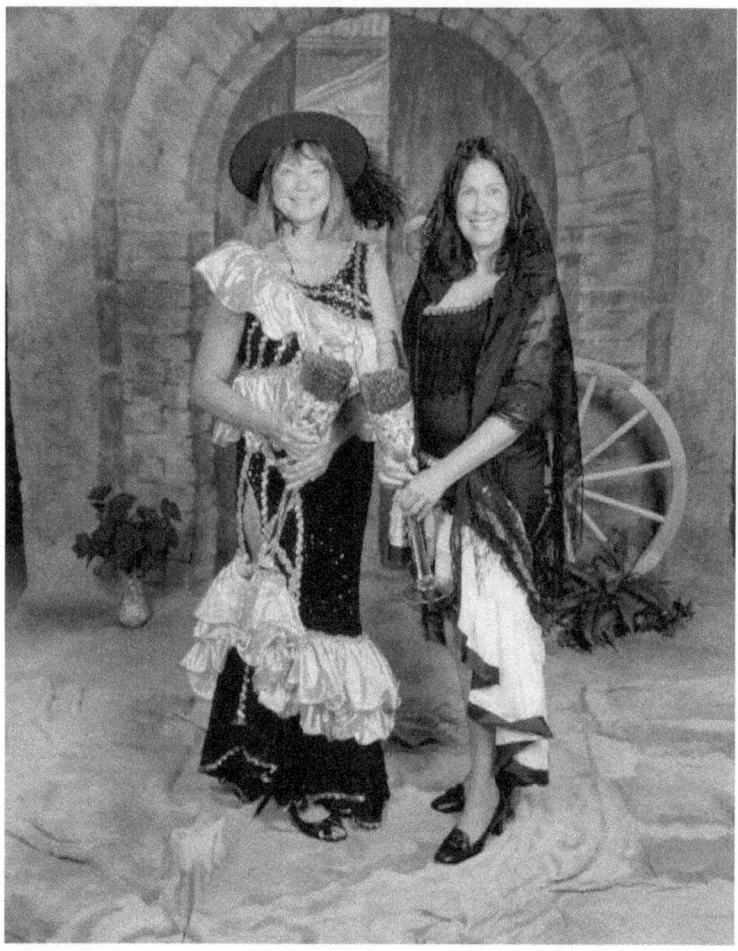

Photo 6 – The first common beans were domesticated about 7,000 years ago in Peru and southern Mexico. Here's a toast to the nutritional boost of the mighty bean!

The Beneficent Bean and the Rest of the Clan of Legumes

Beneficent *adj* generous; conferring blessings. What better adjective to describe beans and legumes? You may not realize that beans are a vegetable, a vegetable which gives us the gift of more fiber and protein than any other. In addition, they confer the blessings of key nutrients often lacking in our diets, including potassium, manganese, copper, magnesium, folate, and iron. Only ½ cup of most beans provides better than 20% of your daily value of folate and protein. Folate helps the body form red blood cells and may reduce the risk of birth defects. Fiber helps reduce the risk of heart disease and certain cancers, and helps maintain a healthy intestinal tract. That same serving of beans also provides 10 to 19% of our daily value of each of the following:

Manganese – helps us build bones and metabolize protein, fat, and carbohydrates.

Protein – essential for growth and maintenance of bones and muscle.

Magnesium – needed for building bone and releasing energy from our muscles.

Copper – essential for iron absorption and efficient use of oxygen.

Iron – helps us carry oxygen in our blood.

Potassium – helps us maintain a healthy blood pressure.

The 2005 Dietary Guidelines for Americans recommends that we eat at least three cups of legumes, such as beans and lentils, each week. And if you do, you can consider yourself blessed by the Mighty Bean.

Just how long have these blessed beans been around? All of us remember the story of Jack and the Beanstalk. This story dates back to 1860, according to Joseph Jacobs, who wrote <u>English Fairy Tales</u> (New York and London: G. P. Putnam's Sons and David Nutt, 1898). Joseph recalled a tale told to him in Australia around 1860, which he later retold in this book.

This date, however, merely scratches the surface of the history of beans. From the royal tombs of ancient Egypt to the classical Greece of Homer's Iliad to the Old Testament, beans can be traced back literally thousands and thousands of years. Legumes, in fact, can be traced back more than 20,000 years in some Eastern cultures, and were a dietary staple in the diet of ancient peoples. The first common beans, including the lima bean and the pinta, or cranberry, bean were domesticated about 7,000 years ago in Peru and southern Mexico. Lentil remains from 10,000 years ago were uncovered on the banks of the Euphrates River in what is now northern Syria. Chickpeas were an ingredient in vegetable soup as early as the 7th century BC in Gaul. Chickpeas were also found in Bronze Age deposits in Jericho and Babylon on the far side of the Mediterranean.

The ancient Egyptians are known to have favored lentils - the remains of a paste of lentils were found in 3rd Century BC tombs at Thebes. In addition, a 2nd century BC fresco shows lentil soup being prepared in the time of Ramses II. In ancient Greece, however, lentils were thought of as "poor man's food."

It wasn't long before cultivation and consumption of chickpeas and faba beans spread throughout Europe. Charlemagne, trying to restore productivity to lands ravaged by war, ordered that chickpeas be planted on the pilot farms of his domains. Umberto Eco, the Italian writer and academic, maintains that the cultivation of beans in Europe during the Middle Ages was of enormous importance, saving Europeans from the tragic fate of malnutrition and possible extinction.

Europeans began to be introduced to some of the exotic foods the New World had to offer in the 16th century, among them the common bean. The "common bean" refers to the seeds of many different beans, including the dry varieties that the English called "kidney beans" in order to distinguish them from their Old World cousins. These hardy New World legumes soon became a popular crop in Europe due to their enormous nutritional value and ease in growing and storing them. They soon became a primary food for sailors, which is how the navy bean got its name.

A 16th century author, Gianbattista Barpo, wrote about the health and nutritional benefits of bean consumption in his book, Le Delizie. He even suggested that beans were not only beneficial to the kidneys and spleen, but also maintained that their consumption would enhance male sexual performance. Would any of you with bean-loving husbands like to substantiate his contention?

Although beans were generally seen as a meat substitute for the poor throughout early history, we can credit Catherine d' Medici of Florence for smuggling beans into France when she married Henry, Duke of Orleans, later to become King Henry II of France. In this case, long live the Queen!

During the Great Depression in the United States, and other times of hardship, beans were promoted as a replacement protein, as meat became scarce and expensive. During World War II, the demand for beans increased as they became a staple in the C-rations used by United States servicemen around the world. After the war, dry bean production escalated to assist the United States' food relief efforts in the war-ravaged countries of WW II.

Today, as people become more health-conscious, they are turning more and more to the mighty bean. In MyPyramid, the USDA's recommended eating plan for Americans, beans and peas are the only foods that appear in two different food groups, Meat & Beans and Vegetables. Beans provide a low-fat, saturated fat-free, and cholesterol-free source of protein, making them one of the shining stars in the Meat & Beans category. In addition, their fiber, folate,

The Beneficent Bean

potassium, and antioxidants make them fit into the Vegetable Group just as nicely. So trade your cow for some bean seeds, and get ready to climb the magic beanstalk to better health.

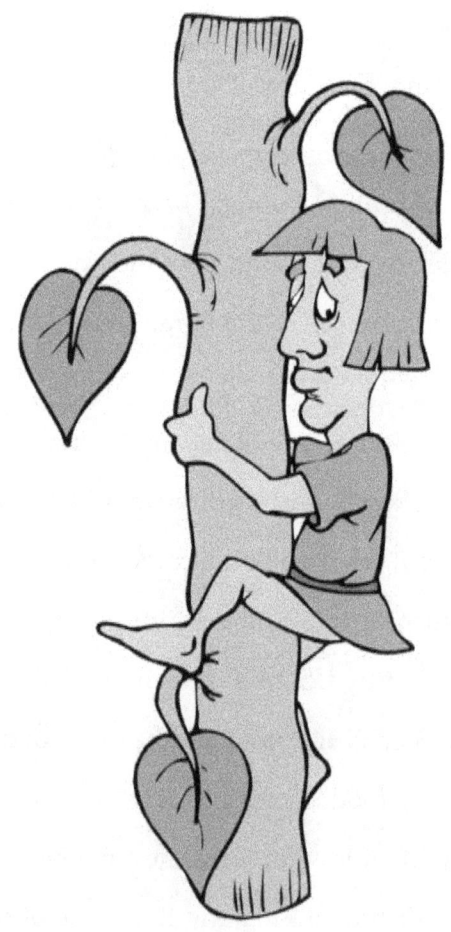

Black Bean and Corn Casserole

- 2 cups chopped onion
- 1 ½ cups chopped green pepper
- 1 14 ½-ounce can tomatoes, undrained and chopped
- ¾ cup green salsa
- 2 teaspoons ground cumin
- 2 cloves garlic, minced
- 2 15-ounce cans black beans, rinsed and drained
- 1 cup canned or frozen corn
- 12 6-inch corn tortillas
- 2 cups reduced-fat Monterey Jack cheese, shredded
- 2 medium tomatoes, chopped
- 2 cups shredded lettuce
- Sliced green onions
- Light dairy sour cream

Combine onion, sweet pepper, undrained tomatoes, green salsa, cumin, and garlic in a large skillet. Bring to a boil, reduce heat, and simmer, uncovered, for about 10 minutes. Add beans and corn.

Place one-third of bean mixture in bottom of a 3 quart rectangular baking dish. Top with 6 of the tortillas, overlapping, and 1 cup of the cheese. Add another one-third of bean mixture and spread out over tortillas. Place remaining 6 tortillas over top, and spread out remaining bean mixture.

Cover and bake in a 350° degree oven for 30 to 35 minutes until heated through. Sprinkle on remaining 1 cup cheese, and let stand 10 minutes. Chopped tomatoes, lettuce, onions, and sour cream are very tasty with this dish. Just sprinkle on top and enjoy! This recipe can be frozen and reheated, but is most visually appealing when first made.

Makes 6 servings.

Black Bean Vegetable Soup

- 1 tablespoon canola oil
- 1 large onion, chopped
- 3 garlic cloves, minced with garlic press
- 3 carrots, finely chopped
- 2 medium sized celery stalks, finely chopped
- 3 teaspoons chili powder
- 1 teaspoon ground cumin
- 4 cups vegetable broth or stock
- 3 cans black beans (15 ounces), rinsed and drained
- 1 ½ cups frozen whole kernel corn
- ¼ teaspoon ground black pepper
- 1 can stewed tomatoes (14.5 ounces)

In a large soup pan, heat oil over medium heat. Add onion, garlic, carrots, and celery, stirring occasionally for about five minutes. When onion is soft, add chili powder and cumin. Cook and stir one minute.

Add vegetable stock, 1 ½ cans beans, corn, and pepper. Bring to a rolling boil.

Puree the tomatoes and remaining 1 ½ cans of beans in a food processor or a blender. Add puree to soup. Reduce heat, cover, and simmer for 10 to 15 minutes, until carrots are tender.

Makes 6 to 8 servings.

Creole Beans and Brown Rice

- 2 cans (14.5 ounces) peeled no salt added diced tomatoes w/juice
- 1 cup uncooked brown rice
- 2 tablespoons canola oil
- ½ cup chopped onion
- 4 cloves garlic, minced
- 1 cup chopped celery
- 1 cup chopped carrots
- 1 cup chopped green and red bell peppers
- 1 tablespoon ground cumin
- 1 tablespoon chili powder
- 1 teaspoon dried basil leaves
- ½ teaspoon cayenne pepper
- 2 cans (15.5 ounces each) kidney beans, drained and rinsed
- 1 can (6 ounces) no salt added organic tomato paste
- 3 tablespoons vinegar
- 1 tablespoon steak sauce or Worcestershire sauce
- 1 teaspoon sugar

Drain juice from tomatoes into a 2 cup liquid measuring cup, and reserve tomatoes for later use. Add water to juice to make two cups. Pour liquid into medium saucepan, add rice, and bring to a boil on medium heat. Reduce heat to low, cover, and simmer 30 minutes or until rice is tender.

Chop all vegetables, combining celery and carrots in a bowl. Heat oil in an extra large skillet or large saucepan on medium heat, and then add onion and garlic. Cook and stir until tender. Add celery and carrots, and cook until crisp-tender, stirring constantly. Add green and red peppers, cumin, chili powder, basil, and cayenne. Cook and stir until peppers are tender.

Add tomatoes, rice, beans, tomato paste, vinegar, steak or Worcestershire sauce, and sugar. Reduce heat to low and heat thoroughly, stirring occasionally.

<u>**Lunch Buddy Notes**</u> – This recipe is very filling, providing 13 grams of fiber.

Makes 8 servings.

Crockpot Bean Soup

- 2 ¼ cups Bob's Red Mill 13 Bean Soup Mix
- 2 30.4-ounce cartons of vegetable broth, plus one 14-ounce can
- 2 cups chopped carrots
- 1 ½ cups chopped celery
- 1 cup chopped onions
- 2 tablespoons tomato paste
- 1 teaspoon Italian seasoning
- ½ teaspoon pepper
- 1 14.5-ounce can diced tomatoes with basil, garlic, and oregano

Combine all ingredients except tomatoes in a large slow cooker, and stir. Cover and cook on low 8-10 hours, or until beans are tender. Stir in tomatoes. Cover and cook on high 10-20 minutes, or until soup is heated through.

Lunch Buddy Notes – We like the unique combination of beans in Bob's Red Mill Bean Soup Mix. Wow, what a powerhouse of fiber – 15 grams per serving (59% of your daily requirement)! You can use any combination of your favorite dried beans in this recipe. If you don't have Italian seasoning, you can put in a pinch of marjoram, thyme, rosemary, savory, sage, oregano, and basil. If you don't have all of these herbs, just put in the ones you do have.

Makes 12 servings.

Italian Bean Soup

- 6 tablespoon extra virgin olive oil
- 2 cups chopped green bell pepper
- 2 cups chopped onion
- 4 garlic cloves, minced with garlic press
- 4 16-ounce cans Great Northern beans, rinsed and drained
- 2 14-ounce cans fat-free, less sodium chicken broth
- 2 14.5-ounce cans diced tomatoes with basil, garlic & oregano, undrained
- 2 tablespoons commercial pesto with basil

Heat olive oil in a large saucepan over medium heat. Add bell pepper and onion. Sauté a few minutes, then add minced garlic.

Cook until onion is tender. Add beans and next three ingredients. Bring to a boil, and then reduce heat. Simmer for 10 minutes, uncovered.

<u>**Lunch Buddy Notes**</u> – Provides 7.2 grams of fiber, 11.9 grams protein, 4.7 mg iron, and 162 mg calcium. This recipe is cholesterol-reducing, quick and easy to make, reheats well, and is one of Susan's favorites.

Makes 8 servings.

Lentil, Barley, and Bacon Soup

- 1 cup lentils
- 1 cup barley
- Olive oil
- 3 to 4 slices of bacon
- 1 cup chopped onion
- 2 cloves garlic, minced
- 2 stalks celery, chopped
- 2 carrots, sliced
- 1 14.5-ounce can diced tomatoes
- Kosher or sea salt and ground black pepper
- Romano or Parmesan cheese

Rinse the lentils and barley well and set aside. Cover the bottom of soup pan with olive oil. Dice three or four slices of bacon, and cook with onions, garlic, celery, and carrots until deep in color, about 15 minutes.

Add tomatoes and stir to coat well. Add lentils and barley and stir to coat well. Add enough water or vegetable broth to cover by a couple of inches, and add salt and pepper.

Bring to a boil, then reduce heat and let simmer until lentils and barley are done, about 40 minutes. Serve with grated cheese.

Makes 8 to 10 servings.

Lunch Buddy Freezer Wraps

- 2 cups uncooked brown rice
- 4 cups water
- 4 15-ounce cans black beans
- 2 15.5-ounce cans pinto beans
- 1 10-ounce can whole kernel corn or 1 ½ cups frozen corn (my favorite is Market Day, sold by the schools)
- 1 10-ounce can diced tomatoes and green chilies
- 16 10" flour tortillas
- 1 pound shredded reduced fat four cheese Mexican cheese or pepper jack cheese

Bring rice and water to a boil in a medium saucepan. Cover and simmer on low for 35 to 40 minutes. When tender remove from heat and cool. This step can be done the day before you plan to assemble the wraps. Simply store rice in a covered container in the refrigerator.

Drain black beans, pinto beans, and corn in a colander and rinse. Transfer to a very large bowl and add diced tomatoes with green chilies. Toss to mix. Add rice and cheese, and gently stir.

If you have a large work area, lay out the tortillas, and divide the mixture evenly among them. If not, just estimate and do a few at a time. If you have extra beans and rice, it's good even without the tortilla, or it could be used as a soup starter. Wrap each one in plastic wrap or aluminum foil. Place several in a large freezer bag, and freeze. Take them out the night before and reheat (about a minute) in the microwave for lunch the next day. And if you like them "hot," you can use pepper jack cheese, or drizzle hot sauce on top to taste. I like them best with fresh salsa.

<u>**Lunch Buddy Notes**</u> – This recipe supplies 13.7g (55%) of fiber, 24.2g (48%) of protein, 45% of calcium, 57% of iron, 66% of thiamin, 61% of niacin, 37% of magnesium, and 110% of folate per serving.* The amazing thing is that there isn't a bite of meat in these wraps. Yet they fill you up, while providing a lot of protein and iron. Now that's a lot of bang for the bean. My son-in-law, a meat lover, tried these and loved them. Susan's husband now eats them as long as she adds chicken and leaves out the black beans. Using canned beans doesn't reduce the nutritional value and greatly speeds up the preparation time. Rinsing the beans cuts down on the sodium. This recipe is pretty easy to make. Cooking the brown rice takes a little time. Once it's done, all you have to do is stir in the other ingredients in a huge bowl, and assemble the lunch wraps. The wonderful thing about this recipe is that when you're finished, you'll have 8 lunches for two in your freezer. If you thaw them first, it only takes a minute or two to heat in the microwave. We like to drizzle hot sauce or salsa on the wraps.

*Percent daily values are based on a 2,000 calorie diet.

Makes 16 servings.

Photo on Back Cover

Penne with a Punch

- 1 14.5 ounce box Barilla Plus Penne Pasta
- 3 tablespoons extra virgin olive oil
- 2 large garlic cloves, minced
- 1 large onion, chopped
- 1 16-ounce jar spaghetti sauce
- 1 15-ounce can black beans, rinsed and drained
- 1 15- ounce can kidney beans
- 1 cup frozen or fresh sweet corn kernels
- 1 pinch chipotle chili powder
- 2 teaspoons ground cumin
- 1 dash hot pepper sauce
- Salt to taste
- Ground black pepper to taste
- 2 tablespoons grated Parmesan cheese

Cook penne pasta in a large pot of boiling salted water until al dente. Drain well. Cook the onion and garlic in olive oil in a large skillet until translucent. Add the spaghetti sauce, black beans, kidney beans, and corn. Mix well. Add the chipotle chili powder, ground cumin, hot pepper sauce, salt, and ground pepper. Stir well. Simmer for 15 to 20 minutes.

Toss pasta with spaghetti sauce, and serve with freshly grated Parmesan cheese.

<u>**Lunch Buddy Notes**</u> – We used Naturally Preferred Organic Mushroom Pasta Sauce, and loved the flavor. The Barilla Plus pasta added 17 grams of protein, 360 mg of ALA Omega 3, and 7 grams of fiber.

Makes 4 to 6 servings.

Provencal Bean Soup

- 1 cup dry pinto beans
- 1 cup dry navy beans
- 3 to 4 quarts water
- 2 medium onions, chopped
- 4 carrots, sliced
- 2 zucchini, chopped
- 3 stalks celery, chopped
- 2 medium potatoes, chopped
- 4 cloves garlic, chopped
- 1 14.5-ounce can diced tomatoes
- ½ cup fresh parsley chopped
- 3 teaspoon kosher or sea salt
- ½ teaspoon ground black pepper
- 1 tablespoon herbs de Provence
- ½ cup small whole pasta
- Freshly grated Parmesan or Asiago cheese

Pick through beans and rinse. In a large stockpot combine all ingredients except pasta and cheese. Bring to a boil, then reduce heat and simmer 2 ½ hours or until beans are tender. Add the small pasta and cook about 10-15 minutes more. Serve with the cheese sprinkled on top.

<u>**Lunch Buddy Notes**</u> – The original recipe called for one or two ham hocks. We preferred to keep this a vegetarian dish. Soaking the beans overnight will cut down on the cooking time. Remember to use a large pot. This soup is a good fiber source and a great way to get your veggies!

Makes 10 servings.

Red Lentil Soup

- 1 ½ tablespoons extra virgin olive oil
- 1 large onion, chopped
- 3 garlic cloves, chopped
- 2 carrots, chopped (1 cup)
- ½ cup chopped fresh or canned tomato
- 1 celery rib, chopped
- 1 ¼ teaspoons ground cumin
- ½ teaspoon salt
- 1 cup dried red lentils
- 4 cups water
- 1 ½ cups chicken broth
- 2 tablespoons chopped fresh parsley

Heat oil in a 4- to 5-quart heavy saucepan over moderately high heat until hot but not smoking. Sauté onion, stirring, until golden, about 5 minutes. Add garlic, carrots, tomato, celery, cumin, and salt and sauté 2 minutes, stirring constantly. Add lentils, water, and broth. Simmer, uncovered. Stir occasionally until lentils are tender, about 20 minutes.

Stir in parsley, then season with salt and pepper.

Lunch Buddy Notes – Recipe adapted from *www.epicurious.com*.

Makes 4 servings.

South of the Border Garlic Vegetable Soup

- Extra virgin olive oil to cover bottom of pan
- 1 medium onion, chopped
- 6 or more of your favorite mushrooms, sliced
- 1 whole head of garlic
- ½ teaspoon red pepper flakes
- 2 teaspoons ground cumin
- 2 teaspoons dried oregano
- 1 15-ounce can diced tomatoes with their juice
- 1 14 or 15-ounce can of Garbanzo beans (chickpeas), drained and rinsed
- 2 carrots, thinly sliced
- 3 cups vegetable broth
- 2 cups baby spinach, chopped
- 2 limes
- 2 avocados

Sauté the onion, mushrooms, garlic, pepper flakes, cumin, and oregano for about 5 minutes. Add the tomatoes, beans, carrots, and broth.

Bring to a boil, then reduce heat. Add the spinach, and simmer the soup until the carrots are tender.

After the soup is ladled into the bowls, squeeze in lime juice and add sliced avocado.

Makes 4 servings.

Tomato, White Bean, and Yellow Squash Stew

- 1 tablespoon extra virgin olive oil
- 2 large yellow onions, chopped
- 2 cloves garlic, minced
- 2 large or 3 medium stalks celery, chopped fine
- 1 14.5 ounce can low-sodium tomatoes, chopped, with juice
- 1 medium-size yellow squash (about ½ pound), sliced thin
- 1 cup fresh or frozen lima beans
- ½ cup dry white wine
- 1 bay leaf
- ¾ teaspoon dried thyme, crumbled
- ¾ teaspoon dried basil, crumbled
- ¾ teaspoon dried marjoram, crumbled
- ¼ teaspoon black pepper
- ⅛ teaspoon cayenne pepper
- 1 can Great Northern or other white beans, drained and rinsed
- 1 teaspoon lemon juice
- 2 tablespoons minced fresh or freeze-dried parsley

Heat olive oil over medium heat for one minute in a heavy 6-quart Dutch oven or soup pot. Add onions, garlic, and celery. Cook, uncovered, for 5 – 8 minutes, until onion and celery are soft.

Add tomatoes, yellow squash, lima beans, wine, bay leaf, thyme, basil, marjoram, black pepper, and cayenne pepper. Stir and simmer, uncovered, for 10 to 15 minutes.

Stir in white beans and simmer 5 minutes more. You can use Great Northern beans, cannellini beans, or navy beans. You can use cooked dried beans, but if you use canned beans, be sure to rinse and drain before adding to lower the sodium.

Add lemon juice and parsley, then stir.

Lunch Buddy Notes – Provides 9 grams of fiber and 13 grams of protein. This is a very tasty stew, which also would be good served over a bed of brown rice. Recipe adapted from Reader's Digest Great Recipes for Good Health, published in 1988.

Makes 4 servings.

Two Bean and Rice Bake

- 4 teaspoons extra virgin olive oil
- 1 tablespoon cumin seeds
- 3 cups onions, chopped
- 2 large garlic cloves, minced
- 1 cup green pepper, diced
- 1 cup petite diced tomatoes with chipotle
- 1 rounded tablespoon chili powder
- 1 ½ teaspoons sea salt
- 16 ounces red beans, drained and rinsed
- 16 ounces black beans, drained and rinsed
- 4 cups cooked brown rice
- 8 ounces reduced- fat Four Cheese Mexican cheese.

Heat oil. Add cumin seeds; cook and stir for one minute. Add onion, garlic, green pepper. Sauté 8 to 10 minutes.

Stir in tomatoes, chili powder, and salt. Bring to a boil. Mix beans and rice, and add to tomato mixture. Sprinkle with cheese.

Bake at 350° for 10 to 15 minutes.

Makes 6 servings.

Vegetarian Chili

- 3 cloves garlic
- 1 tablespoons canola or olive oil
- 2 14.5-ounce cans chunky chili-style tomatoes or stewed tomatoes, undrained
- 1 12-ounce can light beer
- 1 cup water
- 1 8-ounce can tomato sauce
- 3 to 4 tablespoons chili powder
- 1 tablespoon Dijon-style mustard
- 1 teaspoon ground cumin
- ½ teaspoon black pepper
- Several dashes bottled hot pepper sauce
- 3 15-ounce cans pinto beans, white kidney beans, and/or red kidney beans, rinsed and drained
- 2 cups fresh or frozen whole kernel corn
- 1 tablespoon snipped fresh oregano or 1 teaspoon dried oregano, crushed
- ¾ cup shredded cheddar or Monterey Jack cheese (3 oz) (optional)

Cook garlic in hot oil for 30 seconds in large soup pan. Stir in tomatoes, beer, water, tomato sauce, chili powder, mustard, cumin, pepper, and, if desired, hot pepper sauce. Stir in beans and bring to boiling. Reduce heat and simmer, covered, for 10 minutes.

Stir in corn and return to boiling. Reduce heat. Simmer, covered, for another 10 minutes. Stir in fresh oregano, if desired, and top each serving with 2 tablespoons of cheese.

Makes six servings.

Lunch Buddy Notes – Provides a whopping 16 grams of fiber and 17 grams protein; 18% of your vitamin A, 33% vitamin C, 10% calcium, and 18% of your iron for the day.

White Bean Fennel Soup

- 1 large onion, chopped
- 1 fennel bulb
- 3 garlic cloves, minced
- 1 tablespoon extra virgin olive oil
- 5 cups vegetable broth (may use reduced sodium)
- 1 15-ounce can cannelini beans, rinsed and drained
- 1 14.5-ounce can diced tomatoes, undrained
- 1 teaspoon dried thyme
- ¼ teaspoon pepper
- 1 bay leaf
- 3 cups spinach, cut into thin strips

Slice fennel bulb thinly, then crosswise into bite size pieces. Sauté onion, fennel, and garlic in oil in a large saucepan until tender.

Next add broth, beans, tomatoes, thyme, pepper, and bay leaf. Bring to a boil, and then reduce heat. Cover and simmer for about 30 minutes.

Check fennel for tenderness. Remove bay leaf; then add spinach. Cook 3-4 minutes longer or until spinach is wilted.

Makes 5 servings.

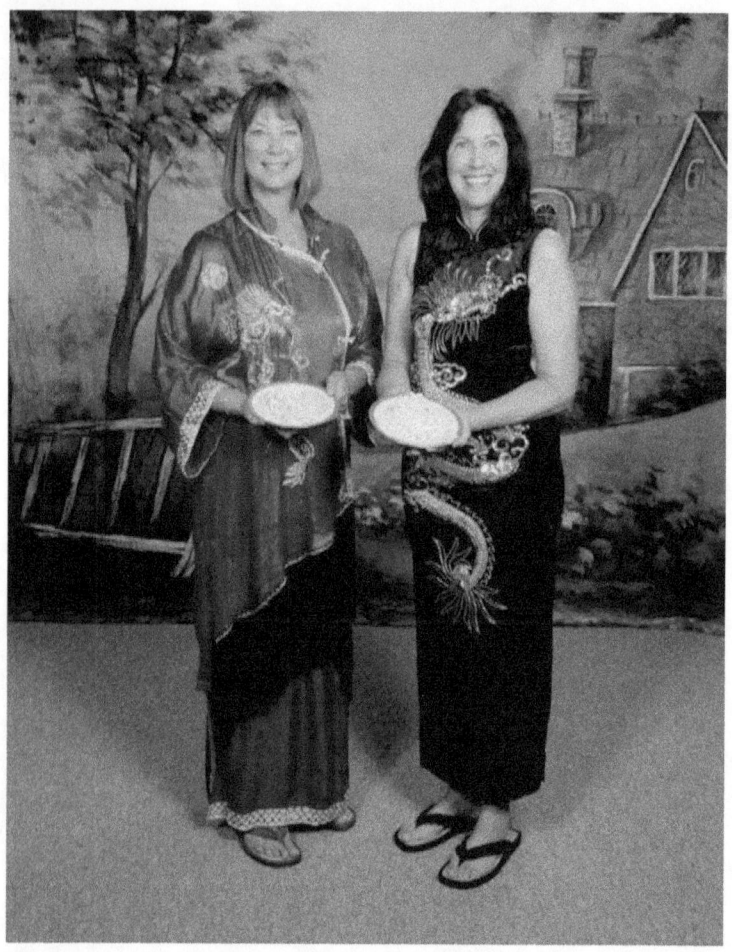

Photo 7 – Think the first pasta was made in Italy? Think again. Actually the Chinese can be credited with inventing the first noodles in 2000 BC.

Pasta Promotion

What do pasta and feet have in common? The ancient method of making pasta was to knead the dough, sometimes for a whole day, with the feet. The Sicilian word "maccaruni", which translates as "made into a dough by force" is thought to be the origin of our word, macaroni. If you had ever kneaded durum wheat, you would most certainly know that force is necessary. Remember "flower power"? Well, the ancient Sicilians knew the meaning of "foot power".

Pasta making as an industry began in Naples, still harnessing "foot power." The pasta maker himself sat on a support while he kneaded the dough with his feet. And you thought your spinning class was difficult. Just think how great your legs might look if you kneaded dough all day … forget jogging and spinning classes … just make pasta!

Although you might think pasta originated in Italy, a well-preserved bowl of noodles over 4,000 years old proved that the Chinese were probably the first to eat noodles, way back in 2000 BC. You might remember a familiar legend that Marco Polo imported the first pasta from China after his travels. Actually we know from several written records that pasta was in Italy before Marco Polo's return. Dry pasta was unknown to the Chinese, who are credited with making pasta from rice flour as early as 1700 BC. In 1295, Marco Polo brought back Chinese dumplings, the first "stuffed pasta", which today has evolved into ravioli and gnocchi.

Italians believe pasta dates back to the ancient Etruscans, who inhabited the Etruria region of Italy from the Iron Age into Roman times. Around 400 BC, they began to prepare a lasagna-type noodle made of spelt. The Romans then made lagane, a kind of lasagna, from a dough of water and flour. Both the Etruscans and the Romans baked their noodles in an oven.

The first Western reference to boiled noodles is in the Jerusalem Talmud of the 5th century CE, according to the American historian, Charles Perry. Evidence exists that by the 10th century, many Arabic sources referred to dried noodles purchased from a vendor. Therefore, credit for the invention of boiled pasta is given to the Arabs. Traders packed dried pasta on long journeys to China. They also carried it to Sicily during the Arab invasions of the 8th century.

How the pasta was eaten is not known, but many old Sicilian pasta recipes still include raisins and cinnamon, introduced most likely by the Arabs. The oldest macaroni recipes are from Sicily: macaroni with eggplant and macaroni with sardines. The Italians most likely were the first to add tomatoes to pasta, creating a marriage made in Heaven.

By the 1300's dried pasta had spread to Genoa, which became a trader and then a producer of dry pasta. Genovese sailors carried the pasta north from Sicily, and to other areas, including Provence and London. Pasta became very popular for its nutrition and its shelf life, and was ideal for long ocean voyages.

By 1400 pasta began to be produced commercially, in shops which hired night watchmen to protect the goods. It was costly to make because (as mentioned earlier) pasta makers had to tread on the dough for nearly a day to make it malleable enough to roll out. Milled durum wheat, or seminola, is granular like sugar, not powdery like other flours. It had to be kneaded for a long time, and then extruded through pierced dies under great pressure, a task accomplished by a large screw press powered by two men or one horse. Yes, you heard right ... pasta was created not only by "foot power," but also by "horsepower"!

Now all of you who have embraced the low-carb or no-carb diets are probably wondering why a chapter is devoted to pasta. Hello, folks. Carboyhdrates are our fuel, providing our bodies with the energy they need for physical activity and for proper organ function. They are an essential part of a healthy diet.

Now, just like you wouldn't want to put watered down gas in your car, you shouldn't put the wrong kind of carbohydrates in your body. Certain easily digested carbohydrates, like white bread, white pasta, white rice, pastries, sugared soda, and other highly processed foods have given all carbohydrates a bad name. These kinds of carbohydrates not only contribute to weight gain. They also increase your risk for diabetes and coronary heart disease.

"The best sources of carbohydrates – fruits, vegetables, and whole grains – deliver essential vitamins and minerals, fiber, and a host of important phytonutrients," as stated on the Harvard School of Public

Health website. So go ahead and enjoy your pasta, as long as it is whole grain. A walk through the pasta aisle in the grocery store is interesting these days. The number of healthy pastas, made from whole grains, nearly equals the number of traditional pastas. Smart Taste, a new white pasta by Ronzoni, contains 6 grams of dietary fiber, 6 grams of protein, and 30% of your calcium for the day. You can even fool your families with this one.

If you decrease your consumption of animal protein by skipping the meat sauce and topping your pasta with a tomato-based, or other healthy sauce, you can enjoy pasta frequently. Be sure to get out your reading glasses and check the list of ingredients on your pasta selection. You might be surprised at all the healthy nutrients inside that box.

Angel Hair with Fresh Herbs and Roma Tomatoes

- 6 ounces whole grain or whole wheat Angel Hair pasta
- ½ cup extra virgin olive oil
- 1 large clove of garlic
- 1 large bell pepper, diced in 1 ½" pieces
- 8 fresh Roma tomatoes, diced
- 1 cup hot pasta water
- Small bunch of fresh herbs, such as chives, basil, parsley oregano, or mint, chopped

Cook pasta according to the package directions and drain, reserving about a cup of pasta water. Heat the olive oil in skillet, and sauté the garlic and bell pepper.

Place the pasta in a serving bowl or if serving the next day, put in a container that has a lid. Toss the fresh diced Roma's, the pasta water, and the olive oil with the herbs.

Lunch Buddy Notes – One Roma gives you 40% of your vitamin C for the day and 20% of your vitamin A. Roma's can be used as regular tomatoes, or for Italian dishes.

Makes 4 servings.

Couscous with Cabbage and Mushrooms

- Extra virgin olive oil
- ¼ onion, chopped
- 1 garlic clove, chopped
- 1 - 2 small carrots, sliced
- 4 - 5 of your favorite mushrooms, sliced
- 1 - 2 cups shredded cabbage
- 1 14.5-ounce can of diced or stewed tomatoes
- 32-ounce container of vegetable broth
- Sea salt
- Black pepper
- 1 cup couscous

Sauté the vegetables and mushrooms in the olive oil for 10 minutes or so.

Add the tomatoes, salt, pepper, and broth. Bring to a boil and simmer until vegetables are tender.

Stir in couscous and cook until thick.

Makes 4 servings.

Marinara Sauce

- 2 tablespoons extra virgin olive oil
- 2 medium onions, chopped
- 1 medium carrot, peeled and finely grated
- 1 teaspoon salt
- ¼ teaspoon red pepper flakes, or to taste
- 1 large can (28 ounces) Italian tomatoes, crushed
- 1 large can (16 ounces) tomato paste
- 1 teaspoon sugar (optional)
- 1 bay leaf (Turkish)
- 2 tablespoons dried whole basil
- 1 teaspoon dried whole oregano
- Pinch fennel seeds
- ¼ teaspoon ground allspice
- 4 cloves garlic, mashed
- Salt or sea salt to taste

In a large pot, heat the olive oil over medium high heat. Add onions and carrot. Sauté until the onions are translucent. Add the salt and red pepper flakes, then the tomatoes and tomato paste. Mix well and bring to a boil. Continue to cook at a simmer.

Add the sugar, herbs, and spices, and simmer uncovered for 30 minutes, stirring occasionally. Add the garlic, and continue to simmer for 30 minutes more or until desired thickness. Add salt to taste. Remove the bay leaf.

Lunch Buddy Notes – This is another daily recipe from Dr. Weil. It's delicious on pasta, rice, or polenta. Tomatoes cooked with oil provide an excellent source of lycopene.

Orange Sesame Couscous

- 2 cups fresh orange juice
- 1 cup chopped red or green bell pepper
- 2 teaspoons sesame oil
- ¼ teaspoon sea salt
- 1 ⅓ cups uncooked whole wheat couscous
- 2 peeled oranges, cut into small pieces
- 6 tablespoons chopped green onions

Combine orange juice, pepper, sesame oil, and salt in a medium saucepan. Bring just to a boil and stir in couscous. Remove from heat and cover.

After five minutes, stir with a fork. Stir in orange pieces and green onions.

Lunch Buddy Notes – Although couscous is generally a refined grain, organic whole wheat couscous is (of course) made from whole wheat, providing 6 grams of fiber and 7 grams of protein per serving.

Makes 4 servings.

Orzo and Mushrooms with Edamame

- 1 16-ounce package of orzo pasta
- 2 tablespoons extra virgin olive oil
- 1 medium onion, chopped
- 2 large cloves garlic, chopped
- 2 stalks celery, chopped
- 8 ounces shiitake mushrooms, sliced
- 8 ounces button mushrooms, sliced
- Sea salt
- Black pepper
- 1 ½ cups vegetable or chicken broth
- 1 ¼ cups low fat milk
- 2 tablespoons cornstarch
- 2 cups edamame
- ¾ freshly grated Parmesan cheese
- ½ teaspoon ground nutmeg

Prepare orzo according to package directions and drain. Place the olive oil in a skillet and over medium heat cook onion, garlic, celery, and mushrooms. Add sea salt and pepper.

In a bowl, mix the cornstarch with the milk and broth, and add to the vegetables in the skillet along with edamame. Bring to a boil, then reduce heat to low and simmer until sauce begins to thicken. Add the cheese and nutmeg and stir to blend. Add more sea salt and pepper, if needed. Stir in orzo and serve.

Makes 6 to 8 servings.

Penne with Roasted Chickpeas, Peppers, and Spinach

- 1½ cups whole grain penne pasta
- Canola or extra virgin olive oil
- 2 cups baby spinach
- 1 16-ounce can chickpeas, drained and rinsed
- 1 red bell pepper, chopped into chunks
- 1 clove garlic, chopped
- ½ teaspoon red pepper flakes, if desired
- Sea salt
- Freshly ground black pepper
- Freshly ground Parmesan cheese

Prepare pasta according to the package directions. Drain and put into large bowl. Then drizzle with a small amount of oil.

Wash the spinach and pat dry. Drizzle oil into skillet and cook chickpeas, red peppers, garlic, salt, black pepper, and red pepper flakes (if using) over medium high heat 10 to 15 minutes.

Remove the peas and peppers to the pasta bowl. Cook the spinach in the same skillet until wilted.

Toss all together and top with freshly grated Parmesan cheese.

Makes 4 servings.

Roasted Roma Penne Pasta

- 9 medium or 7 large Roma tomatoes, seeded and cut into ½-inch slices
- 2 medium or one large zucchini, halved lengthwise and cut into ½-inch slices
- 2 tablespoons extra virgin olive oil
- 4 cloves garlic, minced
- ½ teaspoon sea salt
- ¼ teaspoon black pepper
- 2 cups dried whole-wheat penne pasta (or rotini), about 6 ounces
- 3 tablespoons tomato paste
- ½ teaspoon Italian seasoning (or sprinkle over all)
- ½ cup finely shredded Parmesan cheese
- ¼ cup slivered fresh basil (optional)

Spread tomatoes and zucchini in a 3-quart rectangular baking dish. Combine oil, garlic, salt, and pepper in a small bowl. Drizzle over tomato mixture. Heat oven to 400°, and roast vegetables, uncovered, for 20 minutes, stirring once.

In the meantime, cook pasta according to package directions and drain. Stir tomato paste and pasta into the roasted vegetable mixture. Sprinkle generously with Italian seasoning. Return to oven and bake, uncovered, for 10 to 15 minutes longer (until zucchini looks cooked through).

Stir pasta and vegetable mixture, and divide evenly into four of small bowls, or in Food Saver bags (if freezing). Reheat in microwave, and sprinkle with Parmesan cheese and basil.

Pasta Promotion

<u>Lunch Buddy Notes</u> – This recipe is a modified version of one found in Better Homes and Gardens <u>New Dieter's Cookbook</u>, the cookbook with all the good recipes my husband didn't want to eat. This recipe provides 5 grams of fiber, 12 grams of protein, 32% of vitamin A, 78% of vitamin C, 16% calcium and 16% iron. Overall a very nice nutritional package!

Makes 6 to 8 servings.

Spaghetti with Sun-dried Tomatoes and Peas

- ½ cup sun dried or dried tomatoes, chopped into small pieces
- 1 cup very hot water
- ¼ pound of whole-wheat spaghetti
- 1 tablespoon extra virgin olive oil
- 2 cloves garlic, chopped
- ½ onion, chopped
- Pinch of crushed red pepper flakes
- ½ cup low sodium chicken broth
- 1 cup frozen peas
- ¼ cup fresh basil leaves
- ¼ cup fresh oregano
- Black pepper and sea salt

Soak tomatoes in hot water. Meanwhile, cook spaghetti according to the package directions. While the pasta cooks, sauté garlic, onion, and red pepper flakes in the olive oil in a skillet for 6 minutes.

Drain almost all of the liquid from the tomatoes, leaving just a little. Add tomatoes and reserved liquid, and the chicken broth to the skillet. Add the peas and cook for five minutes. Add the salt and pepper. Chop the herbs, add to the skillet, and remove from heat. Drain the pasta, and divide between two plates or bowls. Top with the tomato and pea mixture. Sprinkle with freshly grated parmesan cheese.

Makes 4 servings.

Tomatoes Stuffed with Vegetable Couscous

- Extra virgin olive oil (a swirl in the pan)
- 1 clove garlic
- Half an onion, chopped
- 1 large carrot, grated or chopped
- 2 cups vegetable broth
- Two large fresh tomatoes with pulp removed and reserved
- 1 cup whole wheat couscous
- Assorted fresh herbs such as parsley, basil, chives, and mint, chopped

Sauté the garlic, onion, and carrot in the olive oil. Add 2 cups vegetable broth, couscous, and the reserved tomato pulp.

Cook until couscous is done. Stir in herbs and fill tomatoes. Serve immediately or can be saved in containers to serve the next day after heating in a microwave.

Lunch Buddy Notes – This recipe was inspired by the fresh herbs and vegetables grown in our garden. You can add any combination of whatever you happen to have on hand. If you like a bigger variety of vegetables, toss in some mushrooms, celery, and green onions.

Makes 2 servings.

Walnut Pasta Toss

- 2 cups whole wheat or whole grain penne pasta
- 3 tablespoons walnut oil
- ½ cup walnuts, roughly chopped
- 1 medium sweet potato, peeled and cut into bites size pieces
- 2 slices red onion, chopped
- 1 clove garlic, chopped
- Sea salt and black pepper
- ½ of a 32-ounce container of vegetable broth
- 1 cup baby greens, Swiss chard, or spinach

Cook pasta according to package directions, leaving the pasta al dente.

Sauté the walnuts in the oil in a skillet for about 10 minutes over medium high heat; then remove to a small dish. Add the sweet potato chunks to the skillet. Cover and cook about 5-10 minutes, removing the lid occasionally to stir. Add onion, garlic, salt, and pepper and continue cooking for 2-3 minutes. Stir in vegetable broth and simmer 5 minutes.

Add the greens, stirring until they are just wilted. Drain the pasta and place in a bowl. Pour the vegetable mixture over the pasta, and add the walnuts. Toss and serve, or refrigerate to share with your lunch buddy the next day!

Makes 2 servings.

Whole Wheat Pasta with Asparagus and Mushrooms

- 5 tablespoons extra virgin olive oil
- 1 pound white or cremini mushrooms, washed, trimmed, and cut into quarters
- Kosher salt
- 5 to 6 medium garlic cloves, minced
- 1 tablespoon sherry vinegar
- 3 tablespoon fresh Italian parsley, chopped
- 1 tablespoon fresh chives, chopped
- 1 tablespoon fresh dill, chopped
- 1 tablespoon fresh rosemary, chopped
- 1 teaspoon coarsely ground black pepper
- 4 ounces freshly grated parmesan cheese
- 1 pound whole wheat spaghetti
- 2 pounds thin asparagus, cut into 2-inch sections

Heat oil in a 12-inch skillet over medium high heat until hot. Add mushrooms, seasoning with ¾ teaspoon kosher salt. Stir to coat, then let cook undisturbed until the liquid released by the mushrooms evaporates and they are deep golden brown, approximately 5 to 7 minutes.

Continue sautéing, stirring occasionally, until most sides are nicely browned, 3 to 5 minutes longer.

Reduce heat to medium and add garlic. Cook just to soften, about 15 to 30 seconds. Add the vinegar and stir, scraping the bottom of the pan, until the vinegar evaporates, about 15 seconds. Remove the pan from the burner and toss in the parsley. Season with more salt to taste, and add chives, dill, rosemary, and coarsely ground black pepper.

Meanwhile, cook pasta as directed in large pot. Drain well, and keep warm. Add asparagus to a large pot of boiling water or steam in the same pan (if using a pasta cooker). Simmer or steam 1 ½ to 2 minutes, until just tender. Drain well.

Add asparagus to mushroom mixture, stirring gently.

Place pasta on plate, covering with mushroom and asparagus mixture. Shave or grate Parmesan cheese on top.

Have some immediately, refrigerating or freezing leftovers to share with your lunch buddy later.

Makes 4 to 6 servings.

Lunch Buddy Notes – This is a fabulous flavor-filled dish, which is fancy enough to serve at a dinner party for Richard Gere, or your own favorite celebrity. It takes a little more time than some of our recipes, but it's definitely worth the effort.

Whole Wheat Pasta with Fresh Herbs

- 6 – 8 Roma tomatoes, peeled and lightly seeded
- 6 - 7 ounces of whole wheat angel hair or spaghetti
- ½ cup extra virgin olive oil
- 1 large garlic clove
- Handful of each of the following:
    - Fresh mint
    - Fresh parsley
    - Fresh basil
    - Fresh oregano
    - Fresh chives

Peel tomatoes by placing them in boiling water for several seconds, then placing them in ice water. Cut them lengthwise, remove most of the seeds, and chop them.

Prepare pasta according to the package directions. Do not overcook! Chop the herbs and garlic, and sauté them with tomatoes in the olive oil.

When the pasta is done, drain well. Top with tomato and herb mixture. Add grated Parmesan if you like. We prefer this dish warmed in the microwave, but it also can be served cold as a salad.

Makes 4 servings.

Versatile Vegetable Hot Recipes

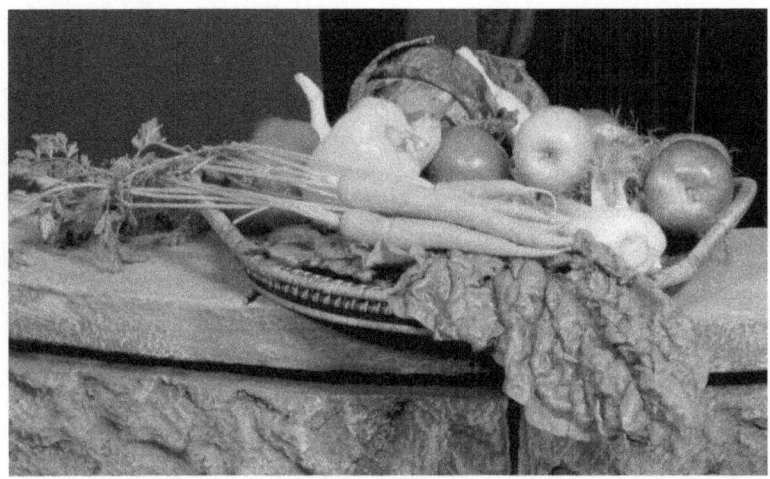

Many vegetables are more nutritious raw; however a few, like tomatoes, are actually better for you once cooked. If you do buy canned, try to find low sodium tomatoes. Vegetables, whether cooked or raw, are one of our most versatile foods. They can be tossed or sautéed together in a multitude of combinations. So load up on your veggies, hot or cold, and enjoy one of our most versatile living foods!

Baked Sweet Potato Slices with Herbs

- 3 sweet potatoes
- ¼ cup Kinloch Plantation Products Pecan Oil
- 1 or 2 cloves garlic, peeled and cut into slices
- Cajun seasoning or herbs de Provence

Preheat oven to 400°. Wash unpeeled potatoes and dry. Cut ends off. Cut potatoes (unpeeled) into chunks or ¼" slices.

Combine pecan oil and peeled garlic slices in a medium bowl. Allow garlic to infuse the oil for 10 minutes.

Remove garlic from oil and discard. Toss potatoes in the garlic-pecan oil.

Place potatoes in a single layer on a baking sheet. Sprinkle with Cajun seasoning or herbs de Provence.

Bake in oven 15 minutes, and then turn potatoes over. Sprinkle other side with seasoning and bake for 15 minutes longer, or until tender.

Makes 4 servings.

Broccoli with Lemon and Dill

- 1 tablespoon extra virgin olive oil
- ½ cup chopped onion or a large leek (white part only)
- 1 clove garlic, minced
- ½ cup reduced-sodium chicken broth
- 1 ½ pounds broccoli, cut into spears
- 1 tablespoon lemon juice
- 1 teaspoon all-purpose flour
- 2 tablespoons snipped fresh dill or 1 teaspoon dried dill
- Sea salt and freshly ground black pepper
- Lemon slices, optional

Heat oil in a large saucepan until hot. Add onion and garlic, and cook about 3 minutes or until tender. Add broth and bring to a boil. Add broccoli, return to boiling; then reduce heat and cover. Cook for 8 to 10 minutes, or until broccoli is tender. Place vegetables in a serving bowl, reserving broth in pan (adding more broth if needed to equal ½ cup).

Combine lemon juice and flour. Stir into broth in saucepan. Keep stirring and cook until thickened and bubbly. Keep cooking an additional minute. Add dill, and salt and pepper to taste. Drizzle sauce over vegetables, and stir lightly to coat. Garnish with lemon slices for visual appeal.

<u>**Lunch Buddy Notes**</u> – Provides 20 % vitamin A, 95% vitamin C, 2 grams fiber, and 3 grams protein. Recipe adapted from Better Homes and Gardens <u>New Dieter's Cookbook</u>.

Makes 6 to 8 servings.

Fabulous Four-Veggie Roast

- 1 tablespoon extra virgin olive oil
- 2 teaspoons soy sauce
- 2 cloves garlic, minced
- 1 teaspoon grated fresh ginger
- 2 large carrots, peeled and bias-sliced into ½-inch pieces
- 1 ½ cups fresh green beans, but into 2-inch pieces
- 5 or 6 small new potatoes (8 ounces), halved
- 1 small onion, cut into wedges
- Freshly coarsely ground black pepper

Combine olive oil, soy sauce, garlic, and ginger in a large bowl. Add carrots, green beans, potatoes, and onion, stirring gently to coat vegetables.

Heat oven to 425°. Place vegetables in a 9x9x2-inch baking pan, spreading evenly. Sprinkle with pepper and roast, uncovered, for 20 to 25 minutes or until just tender, stirring occasionally.

Makes 4 servings.

Healing Cabbage Soup

- 2 tablespoons extra virgin olive oil
- 1 onion, chopped
- 3 cloves garlic, chopped
- 32 ounces low sodium chicken broth
- ½ teaspoon pepper, or to taste
- 1 small head cabbage, chopped
- 1 14.5 ounce can diced or stewed tomatoes

Sauté onions and garlic in the olive oil a few minutes. Stir in chicken broth, pepper if desired, and cabbage. Stir in tomatoes and simmer for 45 minutes or so, stirring often.

Makes 6 servings.

Lunch Buddy Notes – Another great recipe, adapted from *www.allrecipes.com*. We changed this recipe by using low sodium chicken broth instead of the saltier chicken bouillon cubes and water, and eliminated a teaspoon of salt. We also increased the amount of onion and garlic. You won't miss the sodium. This is a great dish to help us get cabbage into our diet, and you'll love it!

Herbed Asparagus with Parmesan Cheese

- 2 pounds thin asparagus, cut into 2-inch sections
- 4 tablespoons extra virgin olive oil
- 1 tablespoon fresh Italian parsley, chopped
- 1 tablespoon fresh chives, chopped
- 1 tablespoon fresh dill, chopped
- 1 tablespoon fresh rosemary, chopped
- 1 teaspoon coarsely ground black pepper
- 4 ounces freshly grated parmesan cheese

Add asparagus to a large pot of boiling water. Simmer or steam 1½ to 2 minutes, until just tender. Drain well. Combine the olive oil, chopped herbs, and pepper and sauté over medium heat in a skillet.

Add the asparagus, tossing gently until heated. Pour the asparagus onto a warm platter, and shave or grate Parmesan cheese over it. Serve immediately, and refrigerate any leftovers.

Makes 6 servings.

Moroccan Vegetable Ragout

- 1 tablespoon extra virgin olive oil
- 1 medium yellow onion, thinly sliced (about 1 ¼ cups)
- One 3- to 4-inch cinnamon stick
- 1 ½ teaspoons ground cumin
- 2 cups peeled and medium diced (½-inch) sweet potatoes
- 1 14- to 16-ounce can chickpeas, drained and rinsed
- 1 14.5 ounce can low-sodium diced tomatoes, with their juices
- 6 tablespoons orange juice, preferably fresh
- 1 ½ teaspoons honey
- 2 cups lightly packed, very coarsely chopped kale leaves (from about ½ pound kale)
- Kosher salt and freshly ground black pepper

In a 5 or 6 quart Dutch oven, heat oil over medium-high heat. Add onion and stir frequently, while cooking, until soft and lightly browned.

Add the cinnamon stick and cumin and cook about a minute, until very fragrant. Add the sweet potatoes, chickpeas, tomatoes with juices, orange juice, honey, and one cup water. Bring to a boil.

Reduce heat to medium low and simmer, covered. Stir occasionally until the sweet potatoes are barely tender, about 15 minutes.

Stir in the kale, cover and continue cooking until wilted, about another 10 minutes. Season with salt and pepper to taste.

<u>**Lunch Buddy Notes**</u> – Recipe modified from one found in the Spring 2008 issue of <u>Dinner Parties</u>. If you like, you can add ½ cup pitted green Greek or Italian olives at the same time you add the chickpeas. And if you don't like olives, simply leave them out. This is excellent served with couscous or our Orange Sesame Couscous recipe on page 199.

Makes 4 to 6 servings.

Oven Roasted Autumn Vegetables

- 1 large sweet potato (10 ounces)
- 1 large fennel bulb (1 pound)
- 8 ounces red potatoes, quartered
- 6 ounces fresh shiitake mushrooms, halved
- 4 large shallots, quartered
- 2 tablespoons walnut oil
- 2 tablespoons balsamic vinegar
- 1 teaspoons coarse salt

Peel sweet potato and cut into small cubes. Cut fennel bulb into wedges.

Toss sweet potato, fennel, red potatoes, mushrooms, and shallots with walnut oil, 1 tablespoon of the vinegar and the salt.

Roast in 425° oven 30 to 35 minutes, stirring a few times. Sprinkle with remaining 1 tablespoon vinegar. Serve warm or at room temperature.

Makes 4 servings.

Raw Roast

- 1 sweet potato, chunked
- 1 onion, chunked
- 1 bell pepper, chunked
- 2 carrots, chunked
- 1 stalk celery, chunked
- 4 cloves garlic, sliced in half
- Sea salt and freshly grated black pepper
- Extra virgin olive oil
- Fresh or dried basil, oregano, mint, and chives chopped

Preheat oven to 425°. Arrange chunked vegetables on a cookie sheet. Sprinkle with salt, pepper, and dried herbs. If you're using fresh herbs, you can sprinkle them on closer to the end of roasting.

Drizzle with oil and toss them lightly with your hands.

Roast in the oven until browned and tender, 30 – 45 minutes.

<u>**Lunch Buddy Notes**</u> – If using fresh herbs chop them all together and sprinkle on the vegetables during the last 5 minutes or sprinkle them on right before serving.

Makes 2 servings.

Red Cabbage with Apple

- 1 tablespoon extra virgin olive oil
- ½ medium onion, chopped (about ½ cup)
- 1 stalk celery, chopped
- 2 thick slices red cabbage, chopped
- 2 stalks Bok Choy, chopped
- 1 apple (not tart), diced
- ¼ cup red wine, optional

Sauté onion, celery, cabbage, and Bok Choy for about five minutes. Add diced apple and cook another 10 minutes, stirring often.

Add the wine, cover, and let simmer for five minutes. Serve warm.

Lunch Buddy Notes – This recipe is another way to get the benefits of the color red … vitamin C, lycopene, and a multitude of antioxidants.

Makes 2 to 3 servings.

Roasted Asparagus with Gruyere

- 2 pounds fresh asparagus spears
- 1 small onion, cut into thin wedges
- 1 small red or yellow sweet pepper, cut into thin strips
- 1 tablespoon extra virgin olive oil
- ¼ teaspoon sea salt
- ¼ teaspoon freshly ground black pepper
- ¼ cup shredded Gruyere or Swiss cheese (one ounce)

Snap off woody bases from asparagus spears, and discard. Scrape off scales if you prefer. In a 15x10x1-inch baking dish, layer asparagus, onion, and sweet pepper. Drizzle with olive oil and toss gently. Spread in a single layer, and sprinkle with salt and pepper.

Heat oven to 400°, and roast about 20 minutes until asparagus is crisp-tender. Just before eating sprinkle with cheese. Let stand 2 minutes to allow cheese to melt.

Makes 6 servings.

Roasted Beets

- Beets
- Onions
- Garlic cloves
- Sea salt and pepper
- Rosemary, fresh or dried
- Extra virgin olive oil

Heat oven to 400°. Wash beets carefully to remove any soil and grit. Cut off the leafy greens, and save them for salad, leaving an inch or so of the stems.

Don't peel the beets. Line a pan with foil and place beets inside. Chunk the onion and add to the beets. Peel and slice garlic cloves, leaving them in big chunks. Add to the beets and onions.

Sprinkle with salt, pepper, and rosemary. Drizzle with extra virgin olive oil.

Bring the foil up around the mixture and roast for 1 ½ hours. Peel the beets and slice to serve at room temperature or heated.

Use any amounts of beets, onions and garlic!

Roasted Ratatouille

- Olive oil nonstick cooking spray
- 3 ½ cups cooked eggplant (1 small)
- 1 cup cubed yellow summer squash or zucchini
- 8 pearl onions, halved
- 1 medium yellow sweet pepper, cut into one inch strips
- 2 tablespoons snipped fresh flat-leaf or regular parsley
- 1 tablespoon extra virgin olive oil
- 2 cloves garlic, minced
- ⅛ teaspoon freshly ground coarse black pepper
- ⅛ teaspoon sea salt
- 2 large tomatoes, chopped
- 1 ½ teaspoons lemon juice

Spray a 15x10x1-inch baking pan with olive oil. Add eggplant, squash, onions, sweet pepper, and parsley to the prepared pan. Stir oil, garlic, sea salt, and pepper together in a small bowl. Drizzle over vegetables and toss to coat.

Heat oven to 450°. Roast vegetables, uncovered, about 20 minutes or until tender and lightly browned. Stir once. Then add tomatoes and lemon juice. Roast 8 to 10 minutes more until tomatoes are very soft and you can see the juice coming out.

Makes 4 servings.

Lunch Buddy Notes – Provides 186% Vitamin C and 19% Vitamin A.

Stuffed Sweet Peppers

- 4 slices firm French bread
- 2 ½ tablespoons rosemary-flavored extra virgin olive oil, divided
- 4 sweet red peppers, divided
- 2 shallots, peeled and chopped
- 8 ounces gouda cheese
- ¼ cup fresh parsley, chopped

Preheat oven to 400°. To make your own flavored olive oil, combine with a twig of fresh rosemary, and allow to infuse for 10 minutes. Remove the rosemary. Tear the bread into small pieces. Heat 1 tablespoon olive oil over medium heat. Add torn bread and sauté, turning until light brown on all sides. Remove from pan and reserve for stuffing mixture.

Cut 2 peppers in half. Scrape out the stem and seeds and discard. Place the 4 halves in a shallow, baking dish cut sides up. Discard the stems and seeds in the remaining 2 peppers. Coarsely chop the peppers into small pieces. Heat 1 tablespoon oil in medium skillet on medium heat, then add peppers and shallots, sautéing until they soften. Cut Gouda cheese into ½ inch cubes.

Toss the sautéed chopped peppers, shallots, toasted breadcrumbs, parsley, and cheese in a large bowl to make the stuffing. Stuff the pepper halves. Brush the top of the pepper halves with remaining ½ tablespoon oil and bake for approximately 30 minutes until tops are light brown.

Makes 4 servings.

Tomato Cabbage Soup with Barley

- 2 tablespoons extra virgin olive oil
- 1 cup chopped onions
- 1 cup chopped celery
- 1 cup chopped carrots
- 2 teaspoons minced garlic
- 2 ½ cups water
- 2 tomatoes, diced
- 1 14.5-ounce can peeled and diced tomatoes with juice
- ⅓ head of cabbage, chopped thin
- 1 32-ounce carton organic chicken broth
- ⅓ cup uncooked pearl barley
- ½ teaspoon ground black pepper

Heat oil, but not to smoking, then add onions, celery, carrots, and garlic. Sauté for 10 minutes or until all vegetables are nearly tender.

Add water, fresh tomatoes, canned tomatoes, cabbage, chicken broth, barley, and ground black pepper. Stir and bring to a boil. Reduce heat to low. Simmer for about an hour, or until barley is tender.

Makes 6 servings, plus one to enjoy after cooking.

Ultimate Vegetable Soup

- ½ cup chopped onion (1 medium)
- 3 cloves garlic, minced
- 1 tablespoon extra virgin olive oil
- 3 14-ounce cans vegetable broth
- 1 cup apple juice
- 1 14.5-ounce can stewed tomatoes, undrained
- 1 ½ cups sliced celery (3 stalks)
- 1 cup thinly sliced carrots (2 medium)
- ⅔ cup coarsely chopped peeled apple (1 medium)
- 1 medium sweet potato, peeled and cut into ½-inch cubes (1 ¼ cups)
- 1 ½ cups shredded cabbage
- 4 ounces fresh green beans, cut into 1 ½–inch pieces (1cup), or 1 cup loose-pack frozen cut green beans
- ½ teaspoon ground coriander
- ¼ teaspoon black pepper

In a 4-quart Dutch oven cook onion and garlic in hot oil about 3 minutes or until nearly tender.

Carefully add the broth, apple juice, tomatoes, celery, carrots, apple, and sweet potato. Bring to boiling; reduce heat. Simmer, covered, for 20 minutes.

Add cabbage, beans, coriander, and pepper. Return to boiling; reduce heat. Simmer, covered, about 15 minutes more or until vegetables are tender.

<u>**Lunch Buddy Notes**</u> – This is truly an ultimate vegetable soup, making the most of an array of produce, and offering just as wide a variety of nutritional benefits. At only 187

calories, a serving provides 5 grams fiber, 5 grams protein, 251% Vitamin A, 35% Vitamin C, 8% calcium, and 8% iron.

Lunch Buddy Notes – Recipe adapted from the Better Homes and Gardens <u>New Dieter's Cookbook.</u>

Makes 8 servings.

Zucchini and Tomato Casserole

- Extra virgin olive oil, about two tablespoons
- 3 small cloves garlic, chopped
- ½ onion, chopped
- 3 cups zucchini with peel on, cubed
- Tomatoes, sliced thin
- Kosher salt
- Pepper

Sauté garlic, onion, and zucchini in olive oil. Spray some extra virgin olive oil in the bottom and sides of a casserole dish. Add a layer of tomatoes, about half the veggie mix, then sprinkle with parmesan cheese, freshly grated. Then add another layer of tomatoes, veggie mix, and parmesan. Bake at 350° for about 30 minutes or until bubbly.

Makes 6 servings.

Quick and Easy Recipes

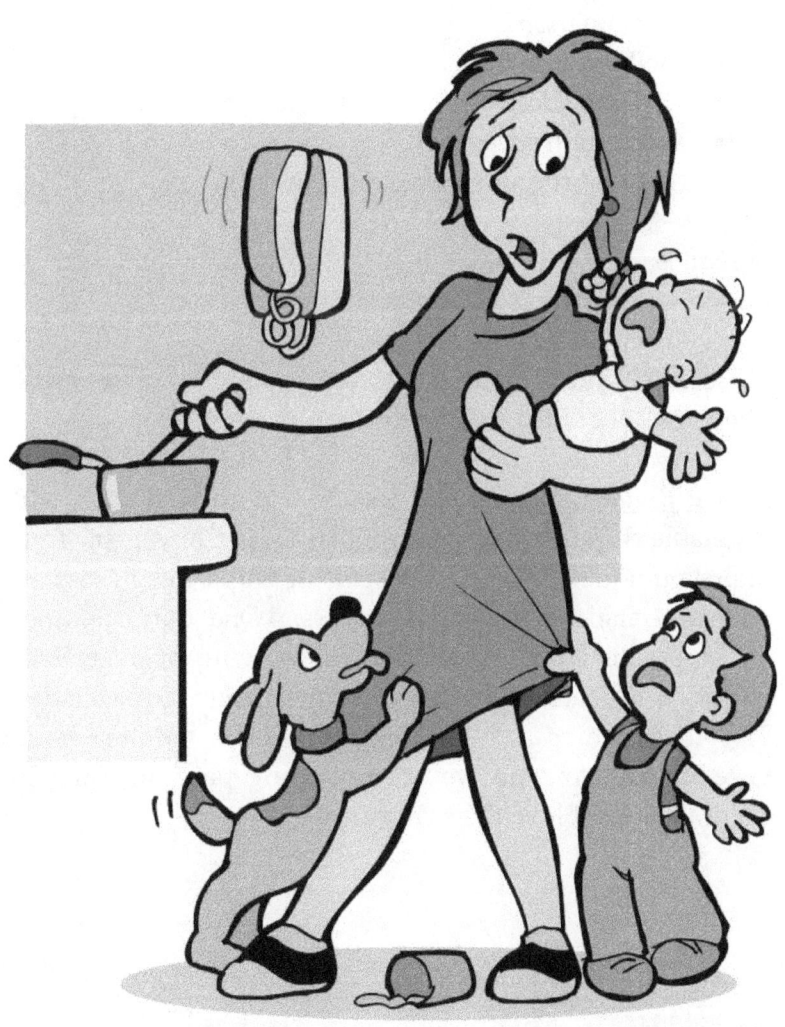

Lunch Buddy Sandwich Wraps

- Hummus
- Romaine, arugula, or spinach leaves, or any combination
- Bell pepper strips
- Tomato slices
- Red onion slices
- Low fat shredded cheese (optional)

Spread each wrap generously with hummus and add the ingredients in order. Wrap up and enjoy!

No cheese? Just go ahead and enjoy them without cheese. They are full of flavor and crunch.

<u>Lunch Buddy Notes</u> – We like to eat these wraps with vegetable chips. In our area, we like Terra Chips best. Terra offers a unique line of exotic vegetable chips, low in sodium, no trans-fats, and delicious flavors. One ounce of their sweet potato chips equals one full serving of vegetables. Sweets and Beets offers 50% of your Vitamin A for the day. Try these chips ... you won't believe you're eating vegetables. (And no we are not being paid anything by Terra ... we just love their chips!)

Quick and Easy Garlic Bread

- Loaf of your favorite bread
- Extra virgin olive oil
- Large garlic clove

Slice the bread and drizzle with the olive oil. Bake in a hot oven, 375° degrees or higher. If you prefer, you can slice a loaf of French bread horizontally and put it under the broiler. When the bread is crispy, remove from the oven.

With one hand, hold a slice of bread with tongs and with other hand, rub the garlic clove gently several times across the bread.

<u>Lunch Buddy Notes</u> – You'll never go back to the loaf of bread with yellow, greasy garlic stuff spread on it! Serve this bread to your family one night, and then bring the leftovers to share with your lunch buddy the next day.

Quick and Easy Recipes

Roasted Red Pepper Hummus

- 2 large cloves garlic, peeled
- 1 15-ounce can chickpeas (garbanzo beans), drained and rinsed
- Juice of one lemon (about ¼ cup)
- Kosher or sea salt and ground black pepper
- Extra virgin olive oil (about two tablespoons)
- ½ cup roasted red peppers (in a jar)

Mince garlic cloves in food processor. Add chickpeas, lemon, salt, and pepper. While processing, add olive oil. Scrape sides of processor and add peppers. Process until peppers are finely chopped.

Put in small bowl, cover and refrigerate.

<u>Lunch Buddy Notes</u> – This recipe can be used in our Lunch Buddy Sandwich Wraps recipe on page 232 or as a dip for pita chips.

Steve's Mango Salsa

- 2 mangoes, diced
- ¼ red onion
- ½ yellow pepper
- 2 cloves garlic, minced
- 2 jalapeno peppers, seeded
- Sea salt
- Juice of 1 lime

Process in a blender on the chop setting, leaving small chunks.

Steve's Salsa

- 2 red tomatoes, diced small
- ¼ red onion, chopped fine
- 2 cloves garlic, chopped fine or pressed
- 2 jalapeno peppers, seeded and diced small
- Sea salt
- Juice of 1 lime

Stir all together.

<u>**Lunch Buddy Notes**</u> – Use gloves when preparing jalapenos! The oil from the peppers can linger on your hands and fingers for days, so be careful! By the way, Steve is Susan's cousin who lives in Texas.

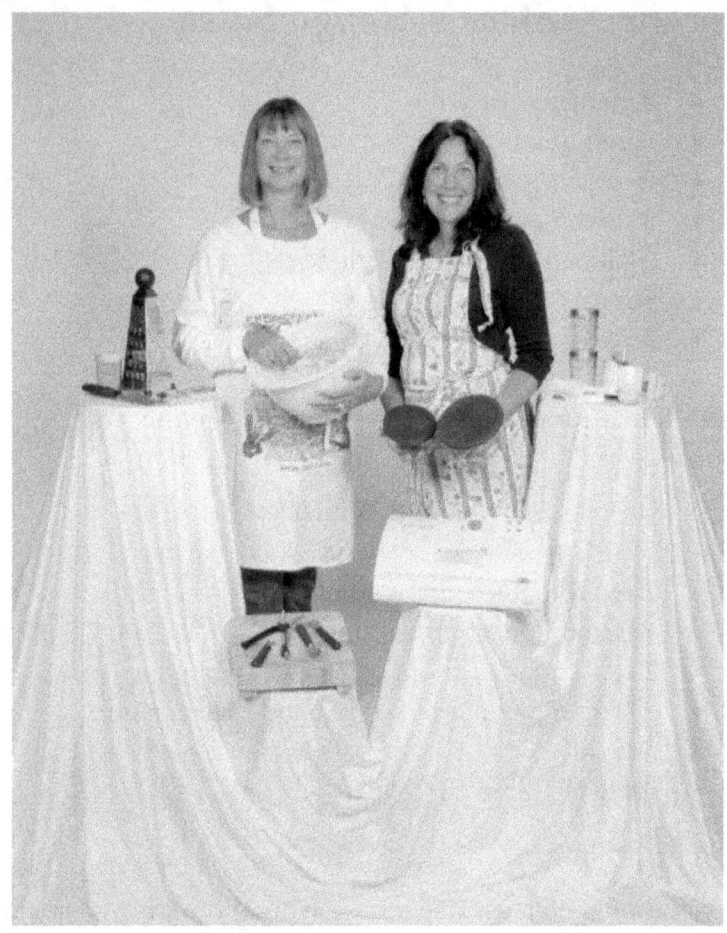

Photo 8 – Anyone can cook from scratch with the right tips, tools, and recipes.

Tips and Tools

Most of us have a buddy or even a group of people we routinely join for lunch. We eat out, order in, eat in our company's cafeteria, or grab something from a vending machine. More often than not, for a variety of reasons, we make choices that taste good, but aren't always good for us. Lunch is often the highlight of our day, both socially and sensually.

Until Susan and I became lunch buddies, I never realized how much I had negatively influenced my previous friends. Remember the strawberry shortcake story? Well when I showed up at the lunch table toting my shortcake (along with my otherwise balanced meal), my friends often returned to the cafeteria line to grab a dessert. Before I became a good lunch buddy, I was a very, very *bad* lunch buddy. For a while I could eat desserts every day and not gain, but many of my friends were not that lucky.

Have you ever noticed the prevalence of obesity in certain departments in your company? If you studied the eating habits of the people in those departments, you would find a great deal of negative influence on each other ... food and candy sitting around, frequent food days, and a contagious attitude of not caring what they eat.

Dan Buettner, author of <u>The Blue Zones: Lessons for Living Longer from the People Who've Lived the Longest,</u> suggests that in order to live longer, healthier lives we need to surround ourselves with the right people. According to Buettner, studies show that if your three best friends are obese, you have a 50 percent greater chance of also being obese.

One study published in the July 26, 2007 issue of the <u>New England Journal of Medicine</u> showed that social networks have contributed to the spread of obesity over the last 30 years. This study also showed that if one member of a social network embraces a healthier diet and exercise habits, the rest of the group will often follow their example.

In the doctor's office where my sister works, pharmaceutical sales reps bring in lunch nearly every day. Whether they bring Steak 'n Shake, Applebee's, Olive Garden, or Quiznos, there's more than enough food to feed the entire staff. My sister, who is diabetic, has had stomach problems for the past few years, and has been unable to eat many solid foods. Yet her coworkers keep urging her to eat with them. They tell her, "One little bite won't hurt you." Frustrated with all this encouragement to eat, she now responds, "It won't help you either." While we should be thinking about food as our fuel, we think of eating as a social event, at home and at work, and we want the people around us to join in on our pleasure.

My husband loves meat. When we go to the grocery store together, he selects the largest, thickest filet he can find and says "Mmmmmmmm," all the way to the checkout line. During dinner, he offers me some of his steak and I respectfully decline. He would like me to join him in his greatest pleasure, and he probably doesn't understand why I don't. Susan and her husband generally eat the same things for dinner; she simply eats less. If she lived alone, she would probably just have a salad. It is clear that we affect the eating choices of those around us, whether coworkers or family.

At an annual dinner where service awards are presented to employees, Susan and her husband Paul joined Jim and me at our table. The guys started talking about our lunches, and Paul asked Jim, "Have you seen what they eat?" Jim simply said, "I've seen it," in a tone of voice which said he couldn't believe anyone would eat that kind of food.

By now, we hope you've tried some of our recipes, and if you have, you know our lunches are delicious. But to someone who is used to a hamburger, fries, and a diet Coke for lunch, like Jim, Summer Garden Quinoa with Strawberry Spinach Salad doesn't look like lunch.

Since that day a couple years ago, we have slowly influenced our families to try some of the food we enjoy so much. Jim tried hummus on pita chips, and said, "Not bad." My son, Mike, even tried whole wheat rotini with marinara sauce and said, "This is pretty good, mom." Susan's husband went to the store and picked up whole wheat buns without being told to buy them. Baby steps in the right direction.

We can influence each other in a positive way. We just have to be persistent and encourage each other to try both new and old foods, some of which we may have previously thought we didn't like. Along this journey to better health, Susan and I have developed some rules, which we call "Lunch Buddy Rules." If you let these rules be your guide, you'll soon be joining us on the successful journey to better health. Bon voyage!

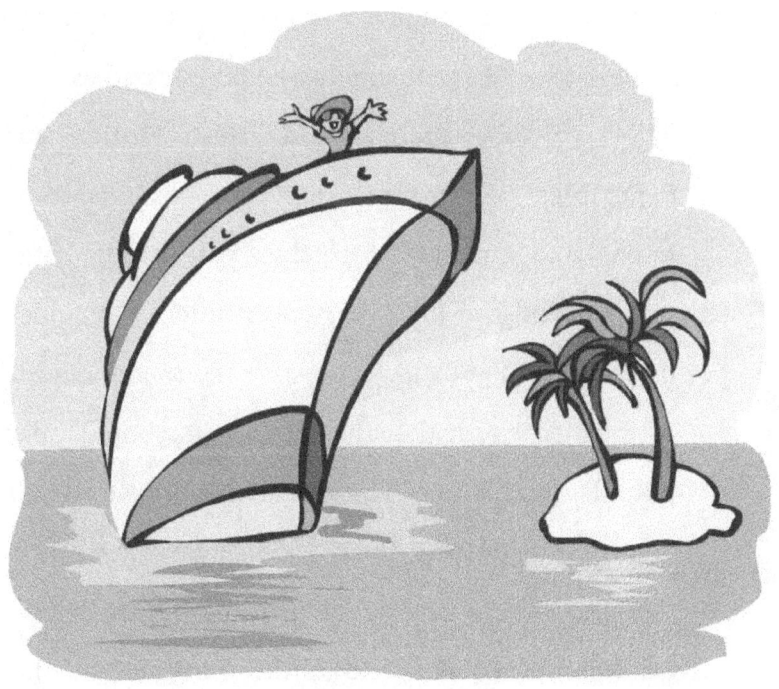

Lunch Buddy Rules

1. **Food has a purpose beyond pleasing our palates.** It is our fuel. If any of you have a high performance car, you are aware that using a higher octane gasoline in your engine will make it run better and last longer. The same holds true for our bodies.

2. **Think whole grains, and fresh fruits and vegetables.** No matter what your goal, the more grains, and fruits and vegetables you eat, the better you will feel and the better you will look. Provided that you don't make poor food choices to supplement your healthy diet, you should shed pounds steadily until you reach your proper weight. A diet emphasizing fresh fruits and vegetables is thought to slow the aging process, improving the condition of our skin, and reducing overall body fat. This diet even improves our breath, as Suzy Cohen advised "Kiss of Death, but Handsome" in Dallas, Texas, whose breath is driving away every woman he dates. Suzy advised this unfortunate guy to stop cooking with so much animal fat, meat, and dairy, and to eat more plant foods, especially parsley.

Plants contain chlorophyll, which is nature's deodorizer. Suzy tells "Kiss of Death" that chlorophyll actually "freshens you from your mouth on down, including your liver, which is crucial." Would any of you Texas ladies like to take on "Kiss of Death," and help him with his new diet?

3. **Eliminate as much meat as you can from your diet.** Dr. Andrew Weil encourages us to decrease consumption of animal protein and increase consumption of vegetable protein. He tells us that animal protein is dense, with more fat and more environmental toxins. These toxins tend to accumulate because animals are higher in the food chain. If you need more reasons not to eat meat, read <u>Skinny Bitch</u> by Rory Freedman and Kim Barnouin and <u>Mad Cowboy: Plain Truth from the Cattle Rancher Who Won't Eat Meat</u>, by Howard Lyman. If it is too difficult to give up meat totally, become a flexitarian (like me). Flexitarians adhere mostly to the vegetarian diet as a healthy lifestyle, but occasionally eat a meal that includes fish, fowl, or meat.

4. **Bring a healthy dish (or dishes) to share, and don't influence each other negatively.** Don't sneak sweets, pop, or fattening chips, and if you lose your will power, **absolutely do not** encourage your lunch buddy to eat these foods too. We have a tendency to feel less guilty about making bad choices if those around us are doing the same. There is probably a psychological term for this phenomenon, and if there isn't, there should be. OK, all you psychologists out there, how about calling it "guilt displacement?"

5. **Overcome your preconceived notions.** Susan thought she didn't like rice or mushrooms and I thought I didn't like beans, especially lima beans. Funny thing is I grew up in Lima, Ohio (pronounced like the bean, not like the capital of Peru). I grew up with canned beans topped with margarine for flavor and didn't like the mushy texture. We used garlic salt instead of fresh garlic when I was growing up. I didn't know what a garlic clove was, so the first time I made spaghetti sauce from scratch, I threw in the whole head of garlic (unpeeled). (Whew, our breath could have made you stop, drop and roll.) You may

Tips and Tools

think you can't cook. Believe me ... if I can learn to cook these foods, you can, too!

6. **Plan and shop ahead.** You can make up menus a week at a time, monthly, or daily.

7. **Cost versus value.** Some of you may hesitate to buy some of the foods we recommend because of their cost. Let's compare a Naked smoothie and a coke. A 15.2-ounce smoothie may cost you around $3.00, while you can buy a can of coke for fifty cents at the grocery store. Which should you buy? While you're shopping, always read labels and think, "What am I getting for my money?" When you buy a coke, you are getting no nutritional value ... basically you are purchasing empty calories. When you buy a Naked Mighty Mango Smoothie, you have to keep in mind the number of servings in each bottle. There are two in the 15.2-ounce size. So right off the bat divide the cost by two, which is around $1.50 per serving. Then read the label ... 130% vitamin A, 250% vitamin C, 300% vitamin E, 10% potassium, 2% calcium, and 2% iron. Look at all the good nutrition you are getting for that extra dollar! A speaker at a seminar I

attended quite a few years ago gave an example of value I will never forget. She talked about the true cost of clothing. Let's say you buy a $35.00 outfit which you wear ten times before it shrinks, fades, or looks so bad you can't bear to wear it. Divide $35.00 by ten. The true cost of that outfit is $3.50. If you spend $100.00 on an outfit and you wear it 200 times, the true cost is fifty cents. Which is the better value? Cost means nothing. Value means everything.

8. **Communicate with your buddy.** If you are sick or forget the food, call your lunch buddy right away. Don't leave a message; call her home phone and her cell phone. She may be able to pull something out of the refrigerator or freezer, or make a quick stop at the grocery store on the way to work. Or if you have a refrigerator/freezer at work, keep a couple extra lunches at work, just in case one of you is ill. Once you begin eating a diet of mostly fruits, vegetables, and grains you may find, as we did, that you don't miss much work. Although I've had a couple colds, I haven't missed a day in more than six years.

9. **Prepare ahead.** If you have a large soup pan, you'll be able to double or triple recipes. Preparing ahead saves time and makes it easy to grab something healthy in the morning, for lunch, or for any meal.
10. **Buy many kitchen gadgets.** They will save you a boatload of time. See our list of Necessary Kitchen Gadgets.
11. **Buy real silverware and plates for your lunch if you have room to store them at work.** If you do, you'll also need dish soap, dish cloths, dish towels, and a dish drainer. Skip this if you don't have access to a sink or storage.
12. **Snack, but choose healthy snacks.** Our favorites include cut vegetables, low-sodium V-8 juice, Naked juices, pomegranate juice, NUT•rition (nuts, of course), or fresh fruit. The Naked juices are like smoothies, with nothing but healthy wholesome ingredients. And here's the scoop on pomegranate juice. According to a recent news story on Good Morning America, Israeli scientists discovered that men who downed just 2 ounces of pomegranate juice daily for a year decreased their systolic (top number)

blood pressure by 21 percent and significantly improved blood flow to their hearts.

13. **Try to maintain healthy eating almost all the time.** Remember me whining in the first chapter about how I didn't have time to make a separate meal for me? Well, a couple years have passed and I have found ways to eat healthy in spite of my family's eating preferences. Here are just a couple examples. If I make spaghetti with meat sauce for the boys (husband and son), I use Ronzoni's Smart Taste pasta for all of us. I use my food saver bags of homemade marinara for my pasta topping. I also make a large salad (minus tomatoes) at the beginning of the week. I add any ingredients which might break down in the salad, such as fruit or tomatoes just before eating. This salad lasts several days. Some of you will be able to educate your families, and they'll follow your good example. I tried that, but my husband soon nicknamed me "The Food Nazi." Do whatever works for you and your family.

Necessary Kitchen Gadgets

1. **Garlic press.** You can do without it if you like to chop, as Susan does. Using a garlic press gives you nice tiny pieces of garlic very quickly. It's even faster to buy a jar of already chopped garlic. You decide ... all methods work.

2. **Cutting boards.** You'll need two ... one for work and at least one for home. If you use a cutting board for meat, don't use it for vegetables and fruits. You need a separate one for each.

3. **Pyrex bowls.** You'll need at least four 2 cup bowls, two 1 quart bowls, and one 1.75 quart bowl. These bowls come with blue lids. We tried one brand and the lids popped off, cracked, or leaked after a few times in the dishwasher. With these bowls, you'll be able to freeze, heat, and serve all in the same bowl. Susan has a large freezer so this is the storage method she prefers.

4. **Soup ladle (one which holds nearly 4 ounces).** Three ladles will fill up your small Pyrex bowl, which is about one serving.

Tips and Tools

5. **Salad tongs.** Keep these at work if you have the room. We make enough salad for at least two days (sometimes three), and use our tongs to fill up our small salad bowls, which we keep at work.

6. **Small slicer.** Pampered Chef makes a nice slicer, called the Egg Slicer Plus, which can be used for strawberries (in salads) or mushrooms. Again, if you like to slice, you don't need this.

7. **Small cheese grater.** We like the Deluxe Cheese Grater made by Pampered Chef. You can even buy a small jar which fits on the grater and stores up to ¾ cup of grated cheese. You can then grate the cheese the night before, and just grab the small jar of parmesan in the morning. Another alternative is to store a cheese grater at work. Voila! Freshly ground parmesan cheese.

8. **Zester.** We like the Pampered Chef Cutting Edge Zester/Scorer, which easily removes peels from citrus fruits, or cuts long strips of peel for garnishing.

9. **Tomato corer and strawberry huller.** Comes in handy. You can easily find one you like just about anywhere.

10. **Juicer.** Extracts juices from citrus fruits.

11. **Sharp knife.** If you can keep this at work, you can just grab a couple pieces of fruit in the morning, and slice it at lunch.

12. **Salad spinner.** Optional, but does a nice job with greens.

13. **Small containers for homemade salad dressing.** We like to use empty pesto or small canning jars. They're a nice size for salad dressing, and best of all, they don't leak.

14. **Food Saver.** Your food saver makes nice flat airtight packages of future lunches. They lie flat in your freezer, and the food stays fresh much longer than if you used Tupperware or other types of storage. Use a permanent marker to label the packages, and if you need to add something to this lunch when serving, jot it down right on the package. For instance, "sprinkle with green onions just before serving," or "add toasted pine nuts." You also may want to add the date prepared. Here's a useful tip ... it is easier to measure your six ladles of soup into a large measuring cup with a spout. Then

pour the soup into a bag and seal. Each bag will contain a lunch for two. This is my favored storage method since I have only a side by side refrigerator/freezer. If purchasing a new Food Saver, I recommend the one with the removable tray. With soups, some is bound to end up in the tray, which can be easily cleaned if removable.

Sample Menu

Breakfast	Steel Cut Oats	4 g. fiber
	Orange	2.6 g. fiber
Lunch	Crockpot Bean Soup	15 g. fiber
	Strawberry Spinach Salad	3 g. fiber
	Red Raspberries (½ cup)	3 g. fiber
Snack	Low Sodium V-8	3 g. fiber
Dinner	Orange Sesame Couscous	6 g. fiber
	Tomato Cucumber Salad	2 g. fiber
	Blueberries (1/2 cup)	2 g. fiber
Total Fiber		40.6 grams

Wow ... 40.6 grams of fiber! See how easy it is to get your fiber when you think about what you are preparing and eating. Since we are not dietitians, we can't give you all the nutritional values of the recipes in this book. You can be assured, however, that the foods we have incorporated in these recipes are among the world's healthiest (and tastiest) foods!

Lunch Buddy Shopping List

Non-Organic Produce
- ☐ Asparagus
- ☐ Avocados
- ☐ Bananas
- ☐ Broccoli
- ☐ Cabbage
- ☐ Corn (sweet, frozen)
- ☐ Kiwifruit
- ☐ Mangos
- ☐ Onions
- ☐ Pineapples
- ☐ Peas (sweet frozen)

Produce, Nuts and Other Essentials
- ☐ Beets
- ☐ Bell Peppers
- ☐ Blueberries
- ☐ Carrots
- ☐ Celery (organic)
- ☐ Fresh Fruits
- ☐ Garlic
- ☐ Greens (organic)
- ☐ Lemons and Limes
- ☐ Mushrooms
- ☐ Onions (non-organic)
- ☐ Orange juice or oranges
- ☐ Parsley
- ☐ Pecans
- ☐ Red onion
- ☐ Tomatoes
- ☐ Walnuts
- ☐ Zucchini

Organic Produce
- ☐ Apples
- ☐ Celery
- ☐ Cherries
- ☐ Grapes (imported)
- ☐ Lettuce
- ☐ Nectarines
- ☐ Peaches
- ☐ Pears
- ☐ Potatoes
- ☐ Spinach
- ☐ Strawberries
- ☐ Sweet Bell Peppers
- ☐ Swiss Chard

Oils, Vinegars, Sauces and Wine
- ☐ Apple cider vinegar
- ☐ Balsamic vinegar
- ☐ Dry sherry
- ☐ Extra virgin olive oil
- ☐ Hot pepper sauce
- ☐ Pecan oil
- ☐ Red wine

Tips and Tools

- Walnut oil

Snacks/Miscellaneous
- Low sodium V-8
- Naked juice drinks
- Parmesan cheese
- Unsalted nuts and seeds
- Terra Chips

Dried, Canned Goods and Cartons
- Canned beans (kidney, Great Northern, pinto, black, Cannellini)
- Canned tomatoes (various kinds)
- Dried beans
- Dried lentils
- Roasted Red Peppers
- Vegetable, Chicken and Mushroom Broth

Whole Grains
- Barley
- Brown Rice
- Pasta (various kinds)
- Quinoa
- Rolled Oats
- Steel Cut Oats
- Whole Wheat Couscous
- Wild rice

Herbs and Spices
- Basil (fresh or freeze-dried)
- Bay Leaf
- Cayenne Pepper
- Chili Powder
- Cinnamon
- Cumin
- Hot pepper sauce
- Kosher Salt
- Marjoram
- Oregano (fresh or freeze-dried)
- Pine Nuts
- Red Pepper Flakes
- Sea Salt
- Thyme

Foods High in Total Antioxidant Capacity (TAC)

Blueberries (wild)	13,427	Per cup
Red Kidney Beans (dry)	13,259	Per ½ cup
Pinto Beans (dry)	11,864	Per ½ cup
Blueberries (cultivated)	9,019	Per cup
Cranberries (whole)	8,983	Per cup
Artichoke (hearts)	7,904	Per cup
Blackberries	7,701	Per cup
Dried Prunes	7,291	Per ½ cup
Raspberries	6,058	Per cup
Strawberries	5,938	Per cup
Red Delicious Apples (w/skin)	5,900	Per apple
Pecans	5,095	Per ounce
Russet Potatoes	4,882	Per potato
Black Plums	4,884	Per plum
Cherries	4,873	Per cup
Black Beans (dry)	4,181	Per ½ cup
Walnuts	3,864	Per ounce
Dried Dates	3,467	Per ½ cup
Ground Cloves	3,144	Per gram
Hazelnuts	2,739	Per ounce
Cinnamon	2,675	Per gram
Broccoli Raab	2,621	Per 85 grams

Tips and Tools

Dried Figs	2,537	Per ½ cup
Red Cabbage (cooked)	2,359	Per ½ cup
Pistachios	2,267	Per ounce
Oregano leaf (dried)	2,001	Per gram

References and Recommended Resources

Books

Chandler, Joanne. Simply Salads. Nashville, Tennessee: Rutledge Hill Press, 2006.

Ody, Penelope. The Complete Medicinal Herbal. New York: Dorling Kindersley, Inc., 1993.

Oxmoor House. The Best of Cooking Light. Birmingham, Alabama: Oxmoor House, Inc., 2004.

Pellman, Phyllis. Fix It and Forget It Lightly. Intercourse, Pennsylvania: Good Books, 2004.

Taste of Home. The Market Fresh Cookook. Greendale, Wisconsin: Reiman Media Group, Inc., 2006.

The Reader's Digest Association, Inc. Foods that Harm Foods that Heal. United States: Reader's Digest Association, Ltd., 1997.

The St. Louis Herb Society. The St. Louis Herb Society Cookbook. Marceline, Missouri: Walsworth Publishing Company, 1994.

Weil, Andrew, M.D. 8 Weeks to Optimum Health. New York: The Ballantine Publishing Group, 1997.

Weil, Andrew M.D. <u>Eating Well for Optimum Health.</u> New York: HarperCollins Books, 2001.

Magazines/Journals/Newspapers

Blackwell, Kelsey. "What You Should Be Eating," <u>Central Illinois Community Health.</u> March, 2008.

Cohen, Suzy, R.Ph., syndicated "Dear Pharmacist" columnist and author of <u>The 24-Hour Pharmacist</u>, "Nature's Deodorizer Can Help Bad Breath," Decatur Herald and Review, October, 2008.

Kady, Matthew. "Food TKO," <u>Clean Eating.</u> Fall 2008.

Planck, Nina. "Superfoods to Know," <u>Parade Weekly Newspaper Supplement</u>, March 30, 2008.

Solan, Matthew. "Mushrooms for a Healthy Heart," <u>Vegetarian Times.</u> September, 2008.

<u>The Herb Companion, 20th Anniversary Issue.</u> November, 2008.

Ward, Bill. "Workers Save by Bringing Bagged Lunches," <u>Decatur Herald and Review</u>. September 22, 2008.

Websites

www.allrecipes.com
www.americanbean.org
www.abcnews.go.com/health
www.bellybytes.com/recipes/couscous.shtml

www.bonappetit.com/
www.bushbeans.com/
www.calorganicfarms.com/
www.centralbean.com/Story_of_Beans.html
www.cyberspaceag.com/kansascrops/wheat/wheathistory.htm
www.dentalplans.com/articles/4933/
www.dolenutrition.com/articleDetails.aspx?RecId=137
www.dried-mushrooms.us/
www.drweil.com
www.ext.colostate.edu/PUBS/FOODNUT/09333.html
www.fitnessandfreebies.com/health/flexitarian.html
www.flaxhealth.com/storage.htm
www.foodreference.com/html/artbeans.html
www.foodreference.com/html/art-rice-history.html
www.fpa-food.org/content/consumers/history.asp
www.fruitsandveggiesmorematters.org
www.geocities.com/sseagraves/historyherbs.htm
www.gicare.com/pated/edtgs01.htm
http://green.msn.com
www.greenbush.net/historyofherbs.html
www.guidetothailand.com/thailand-history/rice.htm
www.health.msn.com/
www.healthcastle.com/
www.herbexpert.co.uk/TheHistoryOfHerbs.html
www.hodgsonmill.com/
www.homecooking.about.com

www.hort.purdue.edu/newcrop/maia/history.html
www.hsph.harvard.edu/nutritionsource/what-should-you-eat/carbohydrates/
www.ific.org/foodinsight/2007/so/processedfoodsfi507.cfm
www.ilovepasta.org/faqs.html#Q3
www.inmamaskitchen.com/FOOD_IS_ART/pasta/historypasta.html
www.johnberardi.com/articles/recipes/brief_history_of_oats.htm
www.keepkidshealthy.com/nutrition/ins_outs_popcorn.html
www.kroger.com/fresh_foods/Pages/dirt_on_organics.aspx
www.mingspantry.com/maitmus.html
www.mushroomlovers.com/Health.htm
www.mypyramid.gov/pyramid/grains.html
http://web.foodnetwork.com
www.nakedjuice.com
www.nationalhealthreview.net/Archive/V02N04/2.asp
www.naturalhealthbenefits.com/health-and-food.html
www.neac.eat-online.net/resources/italy/pasta_history.htm
www.northarvestbean.org/html/schoolbasics.cfm
www.nutritiondata.com/
www.nutsonline.com/driedfruit/sundriedtomatoes/with-olive-oil.html
www.pomwonderful.com/
www.popcorn.org/
www.quinoa-recipes.com/Quinoa_Pages/What_Is_Quinoa.html
www.republicofbeans.com
www.saltinstitute.org
www.sciencedaily.com/releases/2008/01/080108102225.htm

www.thehealthierlife.co.uk/natural-health-articles/nutrition/health-benefits-of-nuts-00841.html
www.thenewhomemaker.com/beansthewonderfulfruit
www.theoi.com/Flora1.html
www.upi.com/Odd_News/2008/02/05/Mac_and_cheese_sales_spike/UPI-90531202243517/
www.veganpeace.com/nutrient_information/recommended_values/daily_values.html
www.vegetablewithmore.com
www.whfoods.com
www.wildrice.org/iwrawebsite/html/wildricehistory.html

Index

A

Afghanistan 42
Alexander the Great 35
allicin 24
Alzheimer's 3, 38, 48
ancient Greeks 42, 93, 95, 104, 106
ancient Romans 36, 95, 103
anise 47
anthocyanin 22, 23, 38, 45
anthocyanocide 38
antibiotics 47
antioxidants 20, 21, 23, 24, 25, 28, 42, 43, 49, 56, 58, 59, 61, 168, 222
Apollo 93, 94
Apples 4, 31, 33, 254, 256
Arabs 192, 193
Archemorus 95
aromatase 115
arthritis 15, 37, 44, 49, 55, 61, 63, 65
Asparagus 33, 207, 219, 223, 254
asthma 15, 44, 63, 65
atherosclerosis 62, 65
avocado 34, 182, 254
Aztecs 145

B

bacteria 30, 38, 106
bananas 20, 24, 35, 51, 56, 77, 143, 254

<u>Barley</u> 37, 62, *121*, 134, *136*, *137*, 146, *147*, 149, *150*, 153, 176, 226, 255
basil 75, 78, 83, 89, 94, 98, 100, 106, 118, 146, *147*, 148, 152, 155, 156, 157, *172*, *173*, *174*, *175*, 196, 198, 202, 204, 205, 209, 220, 255
<u>Bay Leaf</u> 101, 255
Beckman Research Institute 115
beets 19, 20, 23, 24, 35, 36, 61, 63, 224, 232
beeturia 36
Bell Peppers 37, *147*, 254
beta-carotene 35, 39, 52, 65, 102
beta-glucans 114, 116
bioflavonoids 23, 38
<u>Black Pepper</u> 101, 214
Blackberries 37, 77, 256
blood clots 64
blood pressure 23, 36, 44, 55, 97, *127*, 156, 164, 247
blood sugar levels 26, 38, 43, 54
Blueberries 38, 76, 77, 254, 256
boron 58
breast cancer 41, 114, 115
breath freshener 107
broccoli 22, 39, 40, 43, 73, 213, 254, 256
Bronze Age 165
<u>Brown Rice</u> *137*, *157*, *172*, 255
Brussels sprouts 22, 40

Index

C

Cabbage   40, 86, 197, 216, 221, 226, 254, 257
Cachise Indians   144
calcium   35, 39, 47, 50, 61, 64, 66, 88, 100, 104, 105, 106, 108, 111, 119, 175, 178, 187, 195, 203, 228
cantaloupe   24, 41, 42, 80
capsaicin   102
Carboyhdrates   194
cardiovascular health   44, 47, 56
carotenoid phytonutrient   49
Carotenoids   23, 34, 43
Carrots   42, 254
cataracts   37, 41
Catherine d' Medici of Florence   167
Cauliflower   43, 73
Cayenne Pepper   102, 255
Celery   44, 73, 76, 254
Charlemagne   165
Charles Perry   192
Chickpeas   165, 201
China   45, 50, 95, 114, 137, 138, 191, 192
chitin   116
Chives   102
chlorogenic acid   45
cholesterol.   33, 34, 47, 55, 127, 141, 143
Christopher Columbus   52, 61
Cilantro   103
Cinnamon   103, 104, 255, 256
Claudius Galenus   95
colon cancer   36, 38, 48, 54, 56, 61, 63, 65, 115
common bean   166
copper   46, 56, 57, 61, 62, 63, 64, 105, 106, 163

Cortez   145
cradle of civilization   143
cranberries   23, 38, 160
cucumbers   22, 41, 44, 62, 82, 89
Cumin   81, 104, 255
Cupid   93

D

diabetes   15, 65, 104, 127, 134, 194
Dietary Guidelines for Americans   27, 164
digestion   57, 101, 107
digitoxin   98
Dill   71, 104, 105, 213
diverticulosis   26
DNA   38, 50

E

early Celtics   50
Eastern cultures   113, 165
eggplant   23, 45, 46, 193, 224
Egyptians   54, 112, 113, 116, 136, 143, 165
ellagic acid   22, 38, 59
emphysema   41, 64
Environmental Working Group (EWG)   29
enzymes   40, 43, 50
eritadenine   115
esophageal cancer   54
estrogen   58, 115
Etruscans   192

F

Facts and Folklore   29
Fennel   46, 47, 85, 188

Index

Fiber   4, 7, 22 26, 27, 28 33,, 34, 35, 36, 38, 39, 43, 44, 46, 47, 50, 51, 53, 55, 56, 57, 59, 60, 61, 63, 64, 79, 87, 88, 90, 100, 101, 102, 103, 104, 105, 106, 108, 111, 116, 118, 122, 127, 133, 134, 136, 137, 138, 140, 141, 142, 146, 148, 150, 163, 167, 173, 174, 175, 178, 179, 180, 184, 187, 194, 195, 199, 203, 228, 253
flatulence   100, 103, 107
flavanones   55
flavonoids   33, 48, 50, 52, 54, 61
folate   34, 36, 38, 39, 43, 56, 60, 61, 62, 64, 66, 106, 146, 163, 167, 178
folic acid   107
foxglove   98
free radicals   21, 33, 37, 38, 43, 49, 56, 65

G

Galen   96
Garlic   35, 47, 97, 102, 123, 182, 224, 234, 249, 254
Genoa   193
Gianbattista Barpo   166
Ginger   105
glaucoma   97
glucose   141
Grapefruit   49, 74
grapes   22, 23, 48, 49, 58, 77, 80, 254
Great Depression   167
green onions   53

H

Harvard School of Public Health   195
HDL   34
heart disease   15, 22, 38, 49, 61, 97, 114, 115, 127, 133, 134, 163, 194
Hemp   97
hieroglyphics   113
high blood pressure   35
Hippocrates   95, 96
<u>History of Macon County</u>   32

I

immune system   24, 25, 39, 44, 97, 114, 116, 133
Inca Empire   135
indoles   22
Iodine deficiency   110
iron 35, 53, 61, 62, 63, 64, 88, 101, 102, 103, 104, 106, 107, 108, 111, 134, 136, 137, 146, 163, 164, 175, 178, 187, 203, 228
Iron Age   192
Israelites   29, 54
Italy   45, 97, 100, 105, 130, 190, 191, 192

K

kale   40, 50, 76, 217, 218
kidney beans 157, 166, 172, 179, 186
kidney stones   49, 55
King Louis   44
Kiwifruit   50, 254

L

larynx cancer 54
LDL 34, 47
Leeks 51
Legumes 163, 165
LEM 114
Lemons and Limes 52, 254
lentils 4, 75, 146, 164, 165, 176, 181, 255
lentinan 114
limonoids 49, 52
liver 43, 49, 141
Lunch Buddy Rules 242
Lunch Buddy Shopping List 29, 30, 254
lung cancer 43, 114
lutein 22
lycopene 22, 34, 37, 49, 64, 65, 79, 119, 198, 221

M

maccaruni 191
macular degeneration 38, 41, 56
magnesium 47, 59, 61, 62, 64, 66, 100, 103, 105, 138, 163, 178
maitake D-fraction 115
maitake mushrooms 114
manganese 35, 36, 39, 46, 47, 50, 57, 59, 60, 61, 62, 64, 66, 100, 102, 103, 104, 105, 106, 111, 163
Mango 52, 70, 76, 235, 254
Marco Polo 191
melanoma 114
memory 23, 103, 108, 109
Mentha 94
Mesopotamia 143
metabolism 2, 102
Mexico 34, 144, 145, 162, 165

Middle Ages 104, 166
Mint 80, 106
Mushrooms 113, 116, 118, 123, 131, 146, 154, 159, 197, 200, 207
MyPyramid 167

N

Napa cabbage 40, 86
Naples 191
Napoleon years 36
nasunin 45
Native Americans 132, 139
Necessary Kitchen Gadgets 249
Nero 51
New York Medical College 115
niacin 52, 137, 140, 178
nuts 20, 26, 66, 91, 150, 152, 159, 160, 251, 255, 256

O

Oats 140, 141, 254, 255
Omega 3's 39, 61
onions 7, 20, 22, 23, 24, 29, 51, 53, 54, 68, 73, 75, 78, 80, 86, 89, 120, 121, 149, 150, 152, 153, 156, 160, 169, 170, 174, 176, 180, 185, 198, 199, 205, 206, 216, 224, 225, 227, 251, 254
oral cancer 54
oranges 4, 23, 24, 55, 77, 85, 199, 254
Oregano 105, 106, 255, 257
osteoclasts 54
osteopeania 54
osteoporosis 15, 54, 61
ovarian cancer 38, 54, 105

Index

P

Papaya 55
Parsley 95, 107
pasta 63, 78, 106, 108, 118, 179, 180, 190, 191, 192, 193, 194, 195, 196, 198, 200, 201, 202, 204, 206, 208, 209
pattypan squash 61
Pears 56, 254
Persephone 94, 95
Peru 144, 162, 165, 244
phalides 44
Pharaohs 113, 136
phenols 57, 58
phosphorous 47, 62, 64
phosphorus 136, 140
phytonutrients 20, 21, 22, 23, 24, 25, 28, 40, 43, 48, 49, 55, 57, 194
Pilgrims 58
pineapple 24, 56, 77, 254
Plums 57, 256
Pluto 94
Polish women 41
Popcorn 144
potassium 34, 35, 36, 46, 47, 51, 53, 56, 57, 59, 60, 63, 64, 105, 106, 127, 140, 163, 168
Prehistoric civilizations 36
Prometheus 93
prostate cancer 22, 39, 40, 50, 54, 61, 65, 115

Q

quercitin 33, 48, 54
Quinoa 117, 135, 152, 155, 255

R

Radicchio 59, 76
Raisins 58
Rameses III 97
Raspberries 59, 77, 254, 256
red cabbage 40, 222
red onions 53
renal (kidney) cancer 54
resveratrol 48
rheumatoid arthritis 44
rhodopsin 43
riboflavin 136, 140
Romaine Lettuce 59, 76
Rosemary 108, 224
Russian Mennonites 144

S

Sage 109
Salt 72, 78, 109, 110, 124, 146, 179, 198, 213, 255
Sample Menu 253
San Joaquin Valley 58
seminola 193
shiitake mushrooms 114, 118, 120, 121, 122, 159, 200, 219
Spanish and Portuguese explorers 37
spinach 4, 21, 22, 47, 55, 60, 61, 63, 70, 76, 81, 85, 88, 124, 182, 188, 201, 206, 232, 254
stomach cancer 114
Stone Age 56
stroke 15, 38, 48, 49, 62, 134
suforaphane 39, 43
Summer Squash 61
Sweet Potatoes 62
Swiss Chard 63, 64

T

thiamine 140
Thyme 111, 255
Tomatoes 64, 73, 76, 119, 196, 198, 204, 205, 229, 254, 255
Total Antioxidant Capacity (TAC) 21, 256
turnip greens 63

U

ulcers 55, 102
Umberto Eco 165
Unani medicine 96
University of California at Davis 115
University of Minnesota 134
urinary tract infections 23, 38

V

Vitamin A 21, 41, 43, 57, 64, 100, 187, 203, 224, 228, 232
vitamin B 47
vitamin B1 57
vitamin C 21, 22, 23, 33, 34, 35, 36, 39, 41, 43, 44, 47, 49, 51, 52, 54, 55, 56, 57, 59, 60, 64, 187, 196, 203, 214, 221, 224, 228
vitamin K 40

W

Washington 29, 141
Watermelon 65
West Indies 54, 145
white mushrooms 115, 146, 150, 151
whole grain 7, 11, 16, 122, 133, 134, 136, 145, 194, 195, 196, 201, 206, 242
Whole Wheat 126, 143, 207, 209, 255
wild rice 68, 131, 139, 140, 143, 159, 160
wine 48, 71, 81, 82, 83, 100, 119, 126, 129, 131, 221, 254
World War II 167

Y

Yellow Emperor 95, 96
yellow squash 61
yin and yang 96

Z

Zeus 93
zucchini 22, 61, 125, 180, 202, 224, 229

www.ingramcontent.com/pod-product-compliance
Lightning Source LLC
Chambersburg PA
CBHW022108150426

43195CB00008B/321